**NEW DIRECTIONS
FOR MENTAL HEALTH
SERVICES**

Number 9 • 1981

NEW DIRECTIONS FOR MENTAL HEALTH SERVICES

A Quarterly Sourcebook
H. Richard Lamb, Editor-in-Chief

Number 9, 1981

Perspectives on Rural Mental Health

Morton O. Wagenfeld
Guest Editor

Jossey-Bass Inc., Publishers
San Francisco • Washington • London

PERSPECTIVES ON RURAL MENTAL HEALTH
New Directions for Mental Health Services
Number 9, 1981
        Morton O. Wagenfeld, Guest Editor

New Directions for Mental Health Services (publication number
USPS 493-910) is published quarterly by Jossey-Bass Inc., Publishers.
Subscriptions are available at the regular rate for institutions,
libraries, and agencies of $30 for one year. Individuals may
subscribe at the special professional rate of $18 for one year.

Correspondence:
Subscriptions, single-issue orders, change of address notices,
undelivered copies, and other correspondence should be sent to
New Directions Subscriptions, Jossey-Bass Inc., Publishers,
433 California Street, San Francisco, California 94104.

Editorial correspondence should be sent to the Editor-in-Chief,
H. Richard Lamb, Department of Psychiatry and the Behavioral
Sciences, U.S.C. School of Medicine, 1934 Hospital Place,
Los Angeles, California 90033.

Library of Congress Catalogue Card Number LC 80-84291

International Standard Serial Number ISSN 0193-9416

International Standard Book Number ISBN 87589-846-7

Cover design by Willi Baum

Manufactured in the United States of America

Contents

Editor's Notes

Over four hundred years ago, in discussing the several barriers to accurate perception of the world, Francis Bacon noted that we are all prey to the "idols of the cave." Living and working in "caves" (or cities, suburbs, professions, and so forth), we tend to see only that part of the world visible through the cave's small openings. So it was with me until a few years ago. I was the product of a very urban upbringing; only in the past few years, both in the university and in the federal government, have I deeply immersed myself in the problems of rural America's mental health. I am familiar with the range and scope of the problem and am sometimes naively surprised that it is not common knowledge among my fellow academics and health and human services professionals. The clear evidence, however, is that rural America—insofar as its health and human services problems are concerned—suffers from what Leon Ginsberg (1977) has so aptly termed an auditory gap—that is, it simply has problems being heard. This volume is intended to be a corrective in the areas of mental health.

For a variety of reasons, the mental health of rural areas is receiving increasing and necessary attention. The Mental Health Systems Act that was signed into law as this volume was being written mentions the particular needs of rural residents. This is largely an outgrowth of the report of the President's Commission on Mental Health (PCMH) (1978). This document singled out several groups (ethnic and racial minorities, elderly, children, chronic patients, and residents of rural areas) as having been traditionally underserved and in need of corrective attention. The first step in overcoming the auditory gap is developing a consciousness of kind, and this is being done. We now have Washington-based lobbies (such as Rural America, National Rural Center) and professional groups (Association for Rural Mental Health, National Rural Primary Care Association). Professional associations, such as the American Medical Association and the American Public Health Association, have sections or task panels devoted to rural health and mental health problems. Dr. Lucy D. Ozarin of the National Institute of Mental Health (NIMH) has played a major organizing and advocacy role in this area. (See her chapter elsewhere in this volume for discussion of federal advocacy.)

Note: The editor would like to acknowledge the multifaceted assistance of Lucy D. Ozarin, who stimulated his initial interest in studying the problem of rural mental health services delivery and was a source of valuable counsel in the organization and writing of this volume. In a broader sense, the field of rural mental health owes much to her energetic advocacy, parts of which are described in her paper in this volume. Also of great assistance were H. Richard Lamb, the series editor, and Agnes McColley, who did an excellent job of typing the manuscript.

We may ask why this large segment of our population has failed to be heard from in terms of its pressing health and human services needs. To some extent, the explanation is a matter of geography: Rural areas are isolated and their problems and poverty are largely invisible (Harrington, 1962). Additionally, we are victims of another of Bacon's idols—this time, "idols of the tribe"— culturally held beliefs or ideologies. Here, I am referring to a durable and cherished myth in the Western world of the superiority of rural life. Poets, philosophers, and scientists have extolled the virtues of the simple, peaceful, bucolic life and contrasted it with the complexity, stress, and problems of urban existence. But, like many myths of ideologies, this is not the case. Substantial evidence exists that the prevalence rates of many health, mental health, and social problems are substantially higher in rural, as opposed to urban, areas. Discussions of this can be found in Baumheier, Derr, and Gage (1973); Flax and others (1979); Srole (1977); and Wagenfeld (forthcoming).

The problem of high prevalence rates of a variety of health and human services problems in rural areas is compounded by a pervasive poverty (greater than that in urban areas) and chronic shortage of staff that makes the amelioration of these problems difficult. Many rural practitioners have responded to the problematic aspects of their jobs and devised ingenious approaches to their solution. This will be one of the focuses of this volume.

This volume is organized along several dimensions to provide academicians and practitioners with an authoritative source for the state of the art in rural mental health. Mental health problems of rural areas are presented in terms of their theoretical or conceptual, as well as practical, significance. Rural mental health problems are seen in terms of special populations at risk—at the community, state, and federal levels. The chapter by Morton Wagenfeld and Jeanne Wagenfeld (a sociologist and a counselor) sets the stage by considering the problem of the delivery of mental health services in rural areas from a sociocultural perspective. Their main point is that mental disorder—in terms of its definition, treatment, and outcome—is very much a part of culture. Since the definition of disorder is linked to the culture, it is axiomatic (or should be) that services must be delivered in a culturally syntonic manner. Thus, barriers to service delivery either originate with the provider or the client. Providers often deliver their services in terms of an urban, white, and middle-class model, and this is frequently inappropriate for rural populations. Even if services are provided, the values of client groups may militate against their use. In order to aid in the development and delivery of appropriate services, the contributors to this volume sketch out some of the major features of rural life and suggest ways in which service delivery might be improved.

For a number of years, it has been pointed out that a salient feature of rural life has been its poverty, which, in turn, is related to the chronic loss of its most productive populations—young adult and educated. This chronic depopulation has resulted in a disproportionate number of dependent persons — the very young and the elderly — placing a strain on already inadequate health and human services. In other words, one of the sources of stress and social problems in rural areas is this chronic depopulation. Recent demographic data, however, indicate that the long-term trend of outmigration has been reversed.

Rural areas are growing at a faster rate than urban (Economic Development Division Staff, 1978; Schwartzweller, 1979). This is partly a function of a desire on the part of city dwellers to escape the "urban hassle," the increased accessibility of rural areas due to improved highways, and their attractiveness as retirement communities. Most notably, some rural communities — particularly in the mountainous areas in the West — have undergone explosive population growth in connection with energy development. This energy-related growth is an extreme case of community change, but it is an instructive example: Rapid social change has produced disruptions in social arrangements and challenged traditional values for both oldtimers and newcomers alike. These stressors have resulted in a high rate of social problems and an inordinate demand for health and human services. The seeming paradox here is that both loss of population and rapid population growth produce stresses and problems that require therapeutic intervention. Rapid population growth and its consequent human services problems are dealt with in the chapter by Julie Uhlmann, an anthropologist. One of the founders of the Wyoming Human Services Project, she discusses the problems of providing health and human services in energy-impacted areas. She notes that profound changes take place in both the social structure and social relationships in boom towns. The human services delivery system, typically stretched thin even before the boom, is overwhelmed by the epidemic increase in the incidence of health, mental health, and other human services problems. Many of these problems are the same ones that one would expect to see in any community, only at an increased rate, but other problems are unique and related to the stresses of relocation for newcomers and to disruption of established arrangements and values on the part of long-term residents.

Uhlmann details the fiscal and programmatic responses of the human services delivery system in these communities to the challenge of growth and suggests the viability of the model developed by the Wyoming Human Services Project. The project is an example of a creative, multidisciplinary approach to the solving of human services problems in the context of chronic personnel shortages.

Appalachia is, in many ways, prototypically rural: chronically poor, isolated, and with a paucity of health and human services. Steven Giles, a psychologist, describes an ongoing Veteran's Administration program to provide mental health services to Vietnam veterans. Although dealing with a relatively limited population, the program is an example of service delivery that is sensitive to the cultural context of the clients' disorder.

In addition to the attention that the PCMH recommended be paid to rural populations, it also recommended that attention be given to the needs of chronic mental patients. It was recognized that the simple release of patients from mental hospitals into the community serves little purpose except to reduce the census of the institutions. Significant programs of care for these deinstitutionalized patients were needed. Hans Huessy describes some of the historical and contemporary experiences with deinstitutionalization in Vermont.

There has been an increasing recognition that—for the United States in general—a majority of mental health care in both urban and rural areas is rendered in the general medical system (see Hankin and Oktay, 1979; Houpt and others, 1979). As a means of effectively using limited resources, the PCMH's call for a closer integration of the health and mental health systems has particular urgency in rural areas. Carmen Celenza and David Fenton, directors, respectively, of a community mental health and regional health agency in Maine, describe their work in developing an integration of health and mental health services. They trace the evolution of the programmatic effort and discuss the advantages and problems of integration.

It is axiomatic that an effective community mental health effort requires the careful crafting of community support. It may be that the more personalized nature of social relationships in rural areas and the greater visibility of rural agencies and institutions require more attention to the building of support in these areas. The other side of the coin is that these supports result in stronger, more enduring programs. Edwin Fair, who, over a period of over two decades, developed a widely recognized mental health program in a uniquely colorful area of Oklahoma and Kansas, describes the process of building community support.

The Prairie View Mental Health Center in Newton, Kansas has been the recipient of the American Psychiatric Association's Gold Medal Award for making the transition from psychiatric hospital to comprehensive community mental health center. A large part of this transition, as Merrill Raber and Jane Hershberger point out, has involved the extensive development of consultation and education programs. They describe these programs in terms of a matrix, with one dimension being the target population (teachers, clergy, parents) and the other dimension being the type of activity (training, consultation, education, community organization). This conceptualization has resulted in a rich array of programs and activities.

The situation in which community mental health programs are launched in an atmosphere of high expectations and staffed by an enthusiastic and well-funded staff, only to languish for lack of support or be terminated abruptly, is well known to mental health practitioners. P. Vincent Mehmel's paper argues for a process of program development and implementation that he terms the laboratory approach. This approach, which he feels is especially appropriate to rural areas, calls for the piloting of programs with modest fiscal and personnel investments. This approach is advantageous in allowing for—among other things—observing community and staff response, building staff skills, and developing a prestructured, rather than after the fact, evaluation component. Mehmel illustrates the process in terms of several of his center's programs.

Up to this point, the papers focus on mental health problems at the community level. Peter Blouke and David Drachman, working in Montana, consider the problems of mental health at the state level. As planners and evaluators, they note that planning, next to regulation, is the most justifiably maligned occupation of the bureaucracies. One advantage and, presumably, satisfaction in working in a rural state is that the commonly encountered chasm between planners and implementors is reduced. They discuss some of the factors that impact the planning process in a rural state. The new Mental Health Systems Act calls for a closer federal/state partnership, in contrast to the largely federal/local arrangement of the community mental health centers legislation. As state-level staff, they take a rather cautious view of the new arrangement, raising some rather tough questions.

The federal level is the one at which legislation, policy, and funds for mental health and human services most often originate. Lucy Ozarin, who is currently responsible for the rural mental health effort, describes the process of advocacy building at the federal level. Just as the several papers describing the development of programs at the local level stress the importance of building community support, Ozarin underscores the necessity of constituency and resource building at the federal level. In addition to the process of advocacy, she describes some of the outcomes of the effort.

References to the Report of the President's Commission on Mental Health (1978) and to the Mental Health Systems Act have been made in several of the papers. This legislation, much influenced by the report of the PCMH, calls for the development of a second generation of community-based mental health services, special attention to the needs of rural residents and chronic mental patients, and a closer partnership between Washington and the states— issues that are considered in this volume.

Rural mental health centers have developed innovative approaches to services delivery in the face of a high prevalence of disorder and limited fiscal and personnel resources. Hopefully, the Systems Act will become the appropriate institutional response to finally bridge the auditory gap and create a genuinely responsive and equitable services delivery system.

Morton O. Wagenfeld
Guest Editor

References

Baumheier, E. C., Derr, J. M., and Gage, R. W. *Human Services in Rural America: An Assessment of Problems, Policy, and Research.* Denver: Center for Social Research and Development, University of Denver, 1973.

Economic Development Division Staff. "Rural America in the Seventies." *Rural Development Perspectives*, 1978, *1*, 6–11.

Flax, J., Wagenfeld, M. O., Ivens, R. E., and Weiss, R. *Mental Health and Rural America: An Overview and Annotated Bibliography*. Department of Health, Education, and Welfare Publication No. (ADM) 78–753, Rockville, Md.: National Institute of Mental Health, 1979.

Ginsberg, L. "Social Work in Rural Areas." In R. K. Green and S. A. Webster (Eds.), *Social Work in Rural Areas: Preparation and Practice*. Knoxville: University of Tennessee School of Social Work, 1977.

Hankin, J., and Oktay, J. S. *Mental Disorder and Primary Medical Care: An Analytical Review of the Literature*. Department of Health, Education, and Welfare Publication No. (ADM) 78–661. Rockville, Md.: National Institute of Mental Health, 1979.

Harrington, M. *The Other America*. New York: Penguin Books, 1962.

Houpt, J. L., Orleans, C. S., George, L. K., Brodie, H. K. H. *The Importance of Mental Health Services to General Health Care*. Cambridge, Mass.: Ballinger, 1979.

President's Commission on Mental Health. *Report to the President*. Washington, D.C.: U.S. Government Printing Office, 1978.

Schwartzweller, H. D. "Migration and the Changing Rural Scene." *Rural Sociology*, 1979, *44*, 7–23.

Srole, L. "Long-Term Trends in Urban Mental Health: Old Theories and New Evidence from the Midtown Manhattan Restudy." Special Lecture to Opening Day Session, American Psychiatric Association, Toronto, Ontario, May 2, 1977.

Wagenfeld, M. O. "Psychopathology in Rural Areas: Issues and Evidence." In P. G. Keller and J. D. Murray (Eds.), *Handbook of Rural Community Mental Health*. New York: Human Sciences Press, forthcoming.

Morton O. Wagenfeld, professor of Sociology and Health and Human Services at Western Michigan University in Kalamazoo, has done work in mental health delivery systems, worker roles, and psychiatric epidemiology. From 1978–1979 he was on leave at the National Institute of Mental Health, assisting in the development of rural mental health services and research. From 1979–1980, he served as chairperson of the Mental Health Section of the American Public Health Association.

The delivery of mental health services in rural areas may be ineffective
because of client or provider barriers. The nature of these barriers is
discussed, and more culturally appropriate modes of service
delivery are suggested.

Values, Culture, and Delivery of Mental Health Services

Morton O. Wagenfeld
Jeanne K. Wagenfeld

The literature on culture, social structure, and values as independent variables—on the one hand—and mental health as a dependent variable—on the
other—is enormous and spans several disciplines. It is therefore often surpris-
ing that many planners and practitioners fail to appreciate the vast significance of this relationship and have made such simplistic remarks as, "Therapy
is a value-free process," or "You hang your values on the door before you go
into the counseling room."

The aim of this chapter is to examine the relationship of mental health
services to other variables in the community, with particular reference to
sociocultural impediments to the delivery of services in rural areas. This seems
especially relevant in view of the increasing attention paid to rural mental
health in the Report of the President's Commission on Mental Health (1978)
and the Mental Health System Act that has just become law.

Sociocultural Barriers to the Delivery of Mental Health
Services in Rural Areas: Some Conceptual Background

Perhaps the most direct approach to understanding the relationship
between mental health and rural America is to conceptualize it in terms of

sociocultural barriers to the delivery of services. It may be that clients in rural populations do not avail themselves of mental health services (where they do exist) because certain values, such as self-reliance, the nature of man, mistrust of professionals and outsiders, and so forth, militate against getting help for problems of the mind. Client groups may also hold different beliefs about the etiology of mental disorders or have alternative systems of healing and healers. It may also be that the social structure of rural America impedes the establishment of effective delivery systems, or that the nature of mental health services—based largely on an urban, white, middle-class model—is irrelevant to the needs of rural people. In other words, we may have both client and provider barriers. We will discuss both of these possibilities.

Before addressing the issue of cultural barriers, it is first necessary to touch briefly on a number of related issues in rural social structure, mental disorder, and health. More extended discussions can be found in Baumheier, Derr, and Gage (1973), Flax and others (1979), Roemer (1976), and Wagenfeld (forthcoming). Despite a long antiurban tradition in the Western world, there is evidence that rural areas are considerably worse than urban with respect to level of poverty and the prevalence of a wide variety of health and human service problems. The social milieu of these areas serves to exacerbate these problems: Isolation, depopulation, remoteness of health, mental health, and human services, and lagging opportunities for new employment are persistent social problems (Kraenzel and MacDonald, 1971). More recently, some rural areas have experienced profound social problems as a result of burgeoning population growth associated with energy development (Davenport and Davenport, 1979; 1980). A dilemma for rural areas is that these social problems often co-exist with weak or nonexistent social and human services (Flax and others, 1979).

When one talks about social and human services problems in rural areas, it should be pointed out that these may not be rural problems. As noted above, rural areas have more extensive poverty. They also have a higher proportion of the aged and of racial and ethnic minorities, all of whom have been traditionally underserved (President's Commission on Mental Health, 1978). A question that one could ask, then, about the cultural barriers to mental health services is whether we are dealing with ethnicity, rurality, or poverty. It is likely that elements of all three are involved. The Bureau of the Census definition of *rural* is based on population ("an area in which 50 percent or more of the population lives in communities of 2,500 or less"), but the complexity and variety of rural America cannot be captured in this simple, statistical sense. While a neat rural/urban distinction may have had some utility at some point in our history, it is certainly not true anymore. As Hassinger (1976) has noted: "As we examine its characteristics, we see that rural society does not approach homogeneity. The rural segment of this vast nation is differentiated by geographical section, religious and ethnic composition of its population, economic base, and other socioeconomic divisions" (p. 164).

In other words, rural America encompasses whites in such diverse areas as Appalachia and Martha's Vineyard in Massachusetts, Chicanos and Native Americans in the West and Southwest, and both whites and blacks in the South. These are groups with widely disparate values and heritages. Perhaps their only common denominator is that rurality and poverty are largely coterminous.

To the extent that rurality and poverty are closely associated, the large literature on mental health services and the poor is instructive. The results of the landmark study of Hollingshead and Redlich (1958) on the inverse relationship between social class and prevalence of psychiatric disorder and the relationship between class position and kind of treatment are well known. Additionally, Prince (1969), in discussing the problems of psychotherapy among rural poverty populations such as Appalachian whites, pointed out that both the value systems of the poor and certain economic realities present problems for conventional therapy. He argued that economic constraints prevent the poor from utilizing psychotherapy (probably a less valid point today). The time required for results in psychotherapy also presents a problem for the poor, whose time orientation tends to be in the here and now and calls for immediate gratification. Data on the poor in psychotherapy suggest that they tend to be impatient, want immediate results, and expect the therapist to be authoritarian or highly directive. They are also more likely to somatize or to act out their problems. Psychotherapy, as we all know, is a process that takes some period of time. Psychotherapy with the poor is difficult because they are not goal directed; in addition, although the "stuff" of psychotherapy is language, the poor are less verbal and more concrete. Thus the therapy process and relationship are unclear to poor patients and foster a loss of feeling of identity often resulting in greater passivity and dependence. This is clearly counterproductive (Bernstein, 1964). It is a reasonable summary of the literature to say that the poor are poor risks for psychotherapy or refractory to treatment. Excellent summaries of the literature on social class differences in psychotherapy may be found in Frank (1973) and Meltzoff and Kornreich (1970).

To further complicate things it could be argued that certain attitudes, traditions, and values of client populations that run counter to prevailing or majority group norms might militate against the use of existing services or impede the introduction of new services. In addition, client or potential client groups might have a different set of beliefs about the etiology of disorder or have alternative systems of healers.

One could, however, argue that the problem lies with service providers who operate in terms of delivery models that are inappropriate for the social class, region, race, or ethnic group of the clients. The providers, almost always middle class and often white, fail to appreciate the importance of providing culturally syntonic human services. Reul (1974), in writing about barriers to the delivery of services to rural migrants, has outlined a series of client and provider barriers that apply largely to rural populations, particularly the poor.

Perhaps the most pervasive provider barrier is the middle-class nature of the agency itself and its services. Reul also argues that the application procedure, eligibility requirements, agency procedures, and a lack of awareness or sensitivity on the part of the staff are some of the other provider barriers.

More germane to our central concern are the provider barriers of the mental health system—major elements of the human service network. As long ago as 1938, Kingsley Davis, a sociologist, pointed out that the mental health movement was largely a purveyor of white, middle-class values disguised as mental health or medical values. According to Davis, the mental health professional uses psychiatry as a scientific rationalization for conventional middle-class values and goes beyond the illusory goal of mental health to make moral judgments about the whole social system under the "aegis of medical authoritarian mantle."

In the more than forty years that have elapsed since Davis wrote his article, a large literature in psychiatry, psychology, and the social sciences has dealt with the value-laden character of mental health (see, for example, Halleck, 1971; Leifer, 1969; Riessman, Cohen, and Pearl, 1964; Roman and Trice, 1974; Schofield, 1965; and Szasz, 1961). In essence, the argument is that judgments of mental health and illness differ from judgments of physical illness. Values do not enter into the diagnosis of an infection or of diabetes, but the judgment that a person is mentally disordered represents the view that *certain behaviors deviate from a cultural norm.*

This point was made most effectively by Ruth Benedict (1934), the anthropologist who claimed that so-called abnormality is essentially a cultural matter in the sense that those we define as being mentally disturbed function with ease in other cultures. She illustrated this idea by noting that the successful aggressive businessman who is typical of current Western ideals would be considered a serious deviant in other cultures.

The abundant literature suggests that, since value judgments enter into the process of perception, diagnosis, treatment (probability of being accepted into treatment, kind of treatment rendered, and seniority of therapist to whom assigned) and outcome, the value gap between the (largely) white, middle-class service provider and his or her clients is the primary problem. The therapist is essentially an alien to value systems outside of his or her own. Leininger (1971), an anthropologist and nurse, noted that a major problem in community mental health exists in terms of the perceptual and cognitive gap between the professional staff and the lay person's view of the patient's problem, treatment, and rehabilitation. Padilla and Ruiz (1973) illustrated this differential perception of reality in noting that 90 percent of Anglo psychiatric residents associated the patient's hearing voices with psychopathology, in contrast to 16 percent of Mexican-American high school students. Rather than making a diagnosis of auditory hallucinations, it might be more culturally syntonic for therapists to recognize that hearing voices is commonly associated in the Mexican-American culture with a religious calling, something that is hardly unknown in evangelical, Protestant denominations. Related to this is the problem of language. If a value gap exists between therapist and lower class patient, the problem will certainly be exacerbated if one of them speaks a foreign language. The largest foreign language group in our society is the Spanish speaking one, but, even in English speaking subcultures, various slang terms may convey different meanings. Two amusing examples of this were related to us by staff at a local psychiatric hospital who worked with foreign psychiatrists. In the first instance, an adolescent was questioned about his post-hospital plans. When he said that the first thing that he wanted to do was "get wheels," the doctor noted on his chart that he was suffering from delusions relating to his appendages. In the other instance, a patient was telling the psychiatrist that his major problem was that his wife felt that he was "full of shit." The physician prescribed a laxative!

Successful mental health delivery systems require, at the minimum, a shared belief system between providers and clients (see Frank, 1973; Torrey, 1972). In a similar vein, Stenger-Castro (1978) argues that the root cause of mental disorder among Mexican-Americans is generalized estrangement from the dominant Anglo culture and that the major barrier to effective service delivery is ignorance about Mexican-American culture on the part of therapists.

Are certain kinds of therapy less appropriate in rural areas? Mazer (1976) has suggested that rural values seem to militate against the use of long-term, reconstructive therapies. His rural patients in Martha's Vineyard seemed less interested in the maximization of potential or the attainment of happiness than in relief from specific problems. One could question whether this is less a manifestation of a rural/urban difference than of socioeconomic status. In terms of a hierarchy of needs, happiness and personal fulfillment would probably be less salient until the more basic needs of existence are met. The practical utility of Mazer's point, though, remains unchanged.

Oscar Lewis' (1966) famous culture of poverty argument holds that allegiance to the extended family only and a belief in folk healing are dysfunctional in a middle-class, urbanized, and industrialized society. While this may be so in the abstract, the failure on the part of providers to recognize that these practices and beliefs are a reality and serve certain positive functions within the group can be a serious impediment to service delivery. Perhaps illustrative of this value gap and the ethnocentrism on the part of service providers is a tendency to discount indigenous folk-healing practices as nonscientific. Evidence (see, for example, Frank, 1973; Kiev, 1968; Torrey, 1972) indicates that folk healers are frequently effective with their clients because, among other things, they share a common culture and thus a belief system or assumptive world. Leininger (1971) suggested that effective mental health delivery systems must take cognizance of these folk healers and beliefs and integrate them with so-called scientific modalities. Torrey (1970), in discussing mental health services for American Indians and Eskimos, suggested that service providers start with the assumption that mental health services already exist and that they have been at least partially effective. Rather than attempting to supplant these native healers, community mental health practitioners should work cooperatively with them through consultation, education, and planning. Ruiz and Langrod (1976) reported on a program of collaboration between their community health center in New York City and the Puerto Rican community's spiritualists and folk healers. This is certainly in keeping with those basic principles of community mental health that call for working with a community's natural caregivers.

Perhaps less likely to be taken up by service providers is Torrey's (1970) suggestion that secondary prevention should be left to these indigenous therapists since they are part of the culture and already have its social sanction. Similar suggestions about psychiatric consultation to rural Indians were made by Kinzie, Shore, and Pattison (1972).

Padilla, Ruiz, and Alvarez (1975), after outlining the deficiencies of existing community mental health services for Hispanic populations, suggested three alternative models: professional adaptation, family adaptation, and a barrio service center. In the first model, the professional and paraprofessional staff are educated to the needs of the catchment area. The family adaptation model recognizes that the extended family and kinship networks provide important emotional support in times of psychosocial stress and crisis. Finally, in the barrio service center model, the community mental health center reaches out into the community and attempts to help clients with services not directly tied to therapies—jobs, bank loans, and so forth. Although these models were posited for the Hispanic community, it is clear that their implications and application go beyond this group alone. Contained in this model is the recognition that before one can do therapy with a client, more basic needs, such as food or a job must be attended to.

Some final conceptual points relate to the process of seeking help. Medical sociologists are in general agreement that seeking help for physical or emotional problems involves more than the perception of something being wrong followed by the seeking of help. Rather, seeking help is facilitated by a variety of sociocultural and economic variables. Aday (1972) suggested that utilization of health services is a function of three major sets of variables: predisposing, enabling, and need. The *predisposing* included the usual sociodemographic variables, as well as social-psychological factors relating to attitudes toward health care, knowledge of health care information, and psychological and structural stresses. *Enabling* variables stressed economic and organizational factors, while *need* dealt with urgency of symptoms and degree of disability.

In a similar vein, in their national mental health study, Gurin, Veroff, and Feld (1960) pointed out that two sets of variables or factors are involved in the decision to seek help—psychological and facilitating. While psychological factors point toward the use of help as *desirable,* facilitating factors point to the use of help as *available* or *accessible.* If seeking help is seen as a process, then the first step is the definition of a particular problem as within the realm of mental disorder or illness. Here, culturally held beliefs about what is proper or improper are paramount. Having decided that something is a mental health problem, the next decision a person must make is whether or not to seek help. If the decision is made to seek help, then the third step involves where to go for help. In the latter two stages, while values may be involved, it is more likely that structural considerations are more important.

Values of Rural Americans

A fundamental consideration of possible mental health services in rural areas would be that of values. Broadly defined, values refer to culturally held definitions of reality — that is, what is right and proper, the nature of human relationships, and the relationship of human beings to nature. A crucial point about values and value systems is that they are so often taken for granted that they are seldom questioned. For mental health practitioners, this is a crucial (and often overlooked) point.

Given the very heterogeneous nature of rural America, what common values or groups of values can we discern that might impinge on the delivery of mental health services? On the broadest possible level, rural values tend to emphasize several themes: man's subjugation to nature, fatalism, an orientation to the present and to concrete places and things, a view of human nature as basically evil, human activity as being, not doing, and human relationships having their basis in personal and kinship ties. Whether one is talking about Appalachian whites, white residents of Martha's Vineyard in Massachusetts, people of Spanish ancestry, or Eskimos, Native Americans, and blacks, these value orientations are likely to be accurate.* Going from this broad plane, there will be differences among the groups in terms of language, cultural heritage, and historical experience with discrimination and prejudice. If one examines these general rural values, though, one is struck by two points. First, they are similar to Oscar Lewis' delineation of the culture of poverty and often

*The literature on the values of these groups is a field in itself, and that dealing with mental health implications is monumental. Some books with mental health application on Appalachia would be Caudill (1963), Finney (1969), and Weller (1966). Mazer (1976) has written an extraordinary account of life and mental health problems on Martha's Vineyard. An important series of monographs on Latino mental health has been produced by the National Institute of Mental Health (Padilla and Aranda, 1974; Padilla and Ruiz, 1973) and by the Spanish Speaking Mental Health Research Center (Alvarez, 1974, 1975; Miranda, 1976). Kiev (1968) has done an important study of Mexican-American folk healers. On the mental health of blacks, see Thomas and Sillen, 1972; Willie, Kramer, and Brown, 1973. For an interesting account of Native Americans and Eskimos, see Torrey (1970) and Leininger (1971).

antithetical to those of middle-class America. According to Mazar (1976), one of the major stresses for the rural whites on Martha's Vineyard is the very fact that their values are often in conflict with those of the larger society: "The assumptions which guide their lives are challenged daily by what they see on television or read in the newspapers that reach the island. Perhaps more important, their assumptions about life are challenged massively each summer when their values come into conflict with those of their summer visitors, who are many times their number" (p. 41).

While groups in some other locations, more geographically isolated and less popular than Martha's Vineyard, may not witness the same direct confrontation of value systems, the media of mass communication have penetrated to all parts of the country and reduced the isolation of rural America. The conflict between values creates problems that may have significance for the genesis of mental disorders and certainly in the delivery of services. Efforts to alleviate mental disorder and to improve the mental health of communities are likely to fail because the value systems of community residents are somehow wrong with respect to the possibility of salutary change.

It is probably neither the fault of the consumer nor the provider, but rural geography can represent a barrier to the delivery of services. Catchment areas set up for the delivery of community mental health services are based on population, and rural areas are areas of low population density. In many rural areas road networks are poor and public transportation nonexistent, thus increasing spatial isolation and compounding the problem of access. Establishment of satellite clinics has helped to reduce this problem. Hassinger (1976) gave a vivid example of the difficulties created by poor roads in implementing a youth work training program in West Virginia. Roads between some of the hollows were nonexistent and a three mile trip "as the crow flies" meant retracing the route back to the main highway and then travelling over gravel and dirt roads—a distance of twenty-three miles!

In terms of time and effort expended, the major thrust of community mental health has been the delivery of direct services. How do cultural factors influence their use and delivery? Proponents of the culture of poverty perspective would argue that insufficient use of mental health services by the poor (rural and urban) is a function of certain of their attitudes, beliefs, values, or practices. Such people might reject the notion of mental illness as a category, or be suspicious of professionals, or the primacy of extended family ties might preclude going to outsiders for help, or there might be a preference for naturalistic or folk healing techniques. Even if they do get into treatment, their values are incompatible with the goals of psychotherapy and so they are likely to derive less benefit from treatment and to terminate earlier.

An interesting rural/urban contrast in definition and in seeking help for mental disorder was found by Gurin, Veroff, and Feld (1960) in their national survey. A strong gradient existed by degree of urbanization in the definition of a problem in mental health terms: 31 percent in metropolitan areas, in contrast to 20 percent in rural areas. They also found the same urbanization gradient with respect to *readiness for self-referral* — the willingness to seek help for an emotional problem: twenty percent of metropolitan residents and only 9 percent of rural residents had actually used help. A number of respondents indicated that they could have used help but did not do so. When queried on the reasons for not seeking help, the rural/urban gradient showed few differences except in one area. Only 3 percent of metropolitan residents "didn't think that it would help," while 11 percent of the rural residents responded in the same way. Perhaps this is a manifestation of the fatalism that has been characterized as a major rural value.

Perhaps the most useful way to summarize this section is to enumerate the four variables advanced by Torrey to explain the insufficient use of mental health services by Mexican-Americans (and, by implication, other minority, lower class, and rural populations): geographic isolation of facilities, language barriers, class-bound values, and culture-bound values.

Conclusion

In the preceding section, we approached the issue of cultural barriers to the delivery of mental health services in rural areas from two perspectives — dysfunctional values of consumers and class-bound and culture-bound values of providers. Presenting them as opposite poles has probably stereotyped them to an extent. Because rural America is heterogeneous in terms of region and ethnicity, the discussion of rural values has to remain on a level of broad generalization. Because rurality and poverty are so closely related, the problem of service delivery to the poor is applicable in many respects to rural America.

A key term in understanding human behavior is *values*. This has been a focus of the present chapter. Values help shape our perception of reality and serve as anchor points for our lives. But, at the same time, our values, being largely outside of our awareness, are not often examined. It is only relatively recently that the value-laden character of the mental health enterprise has been recognized and attention paid to its implications. As long as adequate mental health care was the province of the urban and the affluent, the value systems of therapist and client were largely coterminous and models of service delivery essentially appropriate. The establishment of community mental health, with its mandate to deliver mental health services to all those in need, has focused attention on the fact that large segments of our population do not operate within the same value system as the majority of service providers.

Old models of service delivery, predicated on a shared assumptive world, have not proven adequate to the task. We have sketched out the dimensions of the problem and suggested some alternative models. In essence, these alternatives recognize the value gap between provider and client and attempt to provide services in a way that will be useful to the client.

Available data suggest that the concept of catchmenting appears to have been successful in helping to deliver mental health services to sections of the population previously inadequately or totally unserved (see, for example, Tischler and others, 1972). The Mental Health Systems Act calls for a more flexible delivery system than that of community mental health centers, but the principle of community-based services remains intact.

Some research on community mental health worker roles and orientations (Jones, Wagenfeld, Robin, 1974; Jones, Wagenfeld, Robin, 1976) suggests that staff in rural community mental health centers differs from its urban counterparts in being focused more strongly on the community dimension of community mental health. Perhaps this is a function of economic realities, the paucity of human services, and chronic staff shortages. We would agree with Milton Mazer (1976), a psychoanalyst transplanted from New York City to rural Martha's Vineyard in Massachusetts, and Edwin Fair, in the present volume, that the therapist in the rural community operates in a milieu totally different from his or her counterpart in the city. In the rural community, the therapist's activities are visible to all, and, much more importantly, he or she is both in and of the community. In this sense, rural community health centers have a unique opportunity to bridge some of these value gaps, overcome some of the cultural barriers, and provide mental health service appropriate to all segments of the population.

References

Aday, L. "The Utilization of Health Services: Indices and Correlates." Paper presented to the Health Services Research and Training Program, Department of Sociology, Purdue University, Lafayette, Indiana, 1972.

Alvarez, R. *Latino Community Mental Health.* Los Angeles: Spanish Speaking Mental Health Center, University of California, 1974.

Alvarez, R. *Delivery of Services for Latino Community Mental Health.* Los Angeles: Spanish Speaking Mental Health Center, University of California, 1975.

Baumheier, E., Derr, J. M., and Gage, R. W. *Human Services in Rural America: An Assessment of Problems, Policy, and Research.* Denver: Center for Social Research and Development, University of Denver, 1973.

Benedict, R. "Anthropology and the Abnormal." *Journal of General Psychology,* 1934, *10,* 59–80.

Bernstein, B. "Social Class, Speech Systems, and Psychotherapy." *British Journal of Sociology,* 1964, *15,* 82–87.

Caudill, H. *Night Comes to the Cumberlands.* Boston: Little, Brown, 1963.

Cutler, D. L., and Madore, E. "Community-Family Network Therapy in a Rural Setting." *Community Mental Health Journal,* 1980, *16* (2), 144–155.

Davenport, J., and Davenport, J., III (Eds.). *Boom Towns and Human Services.* Laramie: University of Wyoming Press, 1979.

Davenport, J., III, and Davenport, J. *The Boom Town: Problems and Promises in the Energy Vortex.* Laramie: University of Wyoming Press, 1980.

Davis, K. "Mental Hygiene and the Class Structure." *Psychiatry,* 1938, *1,* 55–65.

Finney, J. C. (Ed.). *Culture Change, Mental Health, and Poverty.* Lexington: University of Kentucky Press, 1969.

Flax, J. W., Wagenfeld, M. O, Ivens, R. E. and Weiss, R. *Mental Health and Rural America: An Overview and Annotated Bibliography.* Health, Eduation and Welfare Publication No. (ADM) 78-753. Rockville, Md.: National Institute of Mental Health, 1979.

Frank, J. *Persuasion and Healing.* (2d ed.) Baltimore: Johns Hopkins University Press, 1973.

Gurin, G., Veroff, J., and Feld, S. *Americans View Their Mental Health.* New York: Basic Books, 1960.

Halleck, S. *The Politics of Therapy.* New York: Science House, 1971.

Hassinger, E. W. "Pathways of Rural People to Health Services." In E. W. Hassinger and L. R. Whiting (Eds.), *Rural Health Services: Organization, Delivery, and Use.* Ames: Iowa State University Press, 1976.

Hollingshead, A. B., and Redlich, F. C. *Social Class and Mental Illness.* New York: Wiley, 1958.

Jones, J. D., Wagenfeld, M. O., and Robin, S. S. "Rural Community Mental Health Centers: A Unique Breed?" *International Journal of Mental Health,* 1974, *3,* 77–92.

Jones, J. D., Wagenfeld, M. O., and Robin, S. S. "A Profile of the Rural Mental Health Center." *Community Mental Health Journal.* 1976, *22,* 176–181.

Kiev, A. *Curanderismo.* New York: Free Press, 1968.

Kinzie, J. D., Shore, J., and Pattison, E. M. "Anatomy of Psychiatric Consultation to Rural Indians." *Community Mental Health Journal,* 1972, *8,* 196–207.

Kraenzel, C. F., and MacDonald, D. H. *Social Forces in Rural Communities of Sparsely Populated Areas.* Bozeman: Bulletin 647, Montana Agricultural Experiment Station, 1971.

Leifer, R. *In the Name of Mental Health.* New York: Science House, 1969.

Leininger, M. "Some Anthropological Issues Related to Community Mental Health Programs in the United States." *Community Mental Health Journal,* 1971, *7,* 234–241.

Lewis, O. *La Vida.* New York: Random House, 1966.

Mazer, M. *People and Predicaments.* Cambridge, Mass.: Harvard University Press, 1976.

Meltzoff, J., and Kornreich, M. *Research in Psychotherapy.* New York: Atherton Press, 1970.

Miranda, M. R. (Ed.). *Psychotherapy with the Spanish Speaking: Issues in Research and Service Delivery.* Spanish Speaking Mental Health Research Center Monograph No. 3. Los Angeles: University of California, 1976.

Padilla, A. M., and Aranda, P. *Latino Mental Health: Bibliography and Abstracts.* Rockville, Md.: National Institute of Mental Health, 1974.

Padilla, A. M., and Ruiz, R. A. *Latino Mental Health: A Review of the Literature.* Rockville, Md.: National Institute of Mental Health, 1973.

Padilla, A. M., Ruiz, R. A., and Alvarez, R. "Delivery of Community Mental Health Services to the Spanish Speaking Surnamed Population." In R. Alvarez (Ed.), *Delivery of Services for Latino Community Mental Health.* Los Angeles: Spanish Speaking Mental Health Research Center, University of California, 1975.

President's Commission on Mental Health. *Report to the President.* Washington, D.C.: U.S. Government Printing Office, 1978.

Prince, R. "Psychotherapy and the Chronically Poor." In J. C. Finney (Ed.), *Culture Change, Mental Health, and Poverty.* Lexington: University of Kentucky Press, 1969.

Reul, M. R. *Territorial Boundaries of Rural Poverty: Profiles of Exploitation.* East Lansing: Center for Rural Manpower and Public Affairs, Cooperative Extension Service, Michigan State University, 1974.

Riessman, F., Cohen, J., and Pearl, A. (Eds.). *Mental Health of the Poor.* New York: Free Press, 1964.

Roemer, M. I. *Rural Health Care.* St. Louis: Mosby, 1976.

Roman, P., and Trice, H. (Eds.). *Sociology of Psychotherapy.* New York: Jason Aronson, 1974.

12

Ruiz, P., and Langrod, J. "The Role of Folk Healers in Community Mental Health Services." *Community Mental Health Journal*, 1976, *12*, 392–398.

Schofield, W. *Psychotherapy: The Purchase of Friendship.* Englewood Cliffs, N.J.: Prentice-Hall, 1965.

Stenger-Castro, E. M. "The Mexican-American: How His Culture Affects His Mental Health." In A. Ricardo (Ed.), *Hispanic Culture and Health Care.* St. Louis: Mosby, 1978.

Szasz, T. *The Myth of Mental Illness.* New York: Harper-Hoeber, 1961.

Thomas, A., and Sillen, S. *Racism and Psychiatry.* New York: Brunner/Mazel, 1972.

Tischler, G. L., Henisz, J., Myers, J. K., and Garrison, V. "Catchmenting and the Use of Mental Health Services." *Archives of General Psychiatry*, 1972, *27*, 389–392.

Torrey, E. F. "Mental Health Services for American Indians and Eskimos." *Community Mental Health Journal*, 1970, *6*, 455–463.

Torrey, E. F. *The Mind Game.* New York: Emerson Hall, 1972.

Wagenfeld, M. O. "Psychopathology in Rural Areas: Issues and Evidence." In P. J. Keller and J. D. Murray (Eds.), *Handbook of Rural Community Mental Health.* New York: Human Sciences Press, forthcoming.

Weller, J. E. *Yesterday's People: Life in Contemporary Appalachia.* Lexington: University of Kentucky Press, 1966.

Willie, C. V., Kramer, B., and Brown, B. (Eds.). *Racism and Mental Health.* Pittsburgh: University of Pittsburgh Press, 1973.

Morton O. Wagenfeld, professor of Sociology and Health and Human Services at Western Michigan University in Kalamazoo, has done work in mental health delivery systems, worker roles, and psychiatric epidemiology. From 1978 to 1979 he was on leave at the National Institute of Mental Health, assisting in the development of rural mental health services and research. From 1979 to 1980 he served as Chairperson of the Mental Health Section of the American Public Health Association.

Jeanne K. Wagenfeld, a professional counselor, is supervisor of Vocational Evaluation and Assessment at the Jenkins Vocational Rehabilitation Center in Kalamazoo. She has presented workshops dealing with the relationship between values and the provision of client services. In 1980 she was the recipient of the Distinguished Service Award of the Michigan Personnel and Guidance Association.

The recent reversal in migration trends in the United States is generating growth and urbanization in small towns and rural areas nationwide. Although boom towns resulting from energy-related developments in the West may be the extreme case, whatever is learned from studying them should be of use in developing human service programs in other rural areas experiencing growth and change.

Boom Towns: Implications for Human Services

Julie M. Uhlmann

The development of natural resources in the western United States is currently proceeding at a rapid rate as a result of the nation's quest for energy self-sufficiency. Energy-related resources include coal, oil shale, oil, gas, and uranium. The development of these resources involves the construction and operation of new mines, mills, power plants, and processing facilities. Thus, a new industrial life-style is developing in the previously rural, agrarian West.

The industrialization is characterized by a rapid influx of population that results in the generation of boom towns, or energy-impacted communities. Many of these communities have doubled in size in two or three years. The sudden growth frequently has significant negative effects on the quality of life in energy-impacted communities. With experts agreeing that a growth rate over 15 percent per year produces breakdowns in local and regional institutions, a definite challenge to the human service delivery system occurs (Gilmore and Duff, 1975).

This chapter will discuss the effects of energy development on communities in the West, the human needs that arise, and implications for human service delivery strategies in rural areas. Human services include all services provided within a community that are designed to meet the personal and social needs of its residents. In addition to mental health services, this broad definition encompasses areas such as social services, health care, recreation, law enforcement, employment services, seniors' services, youth services, and vocational rehabilitation. A further assumption made in this article is that the human service delivery system in rural communities should be viewed comprehensively.

Characteristics of Preimpact Communities

Over 300 communities in the West have been identified as currently or potentially subject to rapid population growth as a result of the development of energy-related natural resources. Almost two-thirds have populations of less than 2,000. In addition, the communities are widely dispersed geographically. Almost three-fourths are located over 100 miles from a metropolitan area. Interestingly, over one million people live in these communities (U.S. Region VIII Department of Energy, 1979).

Prior to the growth and industrialization associated with energy development, potentially impacted communities exhibit a number of traits that have resulted from out-migration from the nation's rural areas. This depopulation, associated with the mechanization of agriculture, has left rural western communities with few employment opportunities, low tax bases, and near capacity use of existing community facilities.

One implication for human service delivery of these characteristics is that preimpact communities have serious existing needs for human services and few formal resources to meet those needs. For example, a survey of forty critically impacted communities found that 70 percent had no mental health center in the community and over half had no alcohol/drug abuse counseling services or social services office (Uhlmann, 1978). When growth occurs, in addition to providing for the needs of an influx of new residents, rural communities must provide for existing human service deficits (Baumheier, Derr, and Gage, 1973).

Although the human services agency structure may be rudimentary in preimpact communities, many of the human service needs that exist are met informally through families, friends, and neighbors. For many residents, the lack of services is an acceptable trade-off of the rural lifestyle. It is important to note that conditions that outside evaluators may perceive as deficiencies in infrastructure may be acceptable to local residents. Individualistic and personalistic ethics are quite strong in rural western communities.

Population Growth: The Impacting Force

Because of the isolation and small size of rural communities in the West, most of the work force needed for energy resource development must be imported. The size of the imported work force is the central variable influencing population growth. It is related to phase (construction or operation) and type of development. For example, a coal export mine that will produce nine million tons of coal per year would require a peak construction force of approximately 200 and an operating work force around 475. However, a 2,250 megawatt coal-fired electrical generation plant and mine could require up to 3,000 workers during the construction phase and an operating force of 400 (U.S. Department of Housing and Urban Development, 1976).

The primary industrial work force generates a secondary work force composed of support workers in such areas as retail trade, insurance, transportation, government, and human services. As the primary work force increases, the number of support workers also increases.

To forecast total population growth, the size of the primary and secondary work force, the average number of family members associated with each work force, and the percent of workers hired locally must be estimated. Considering all these factors, the work force of 3,000 needed to construct the coal-fired power plant in the example above could generate a total new population of 7,000. Clearly, this would represent significant growth for most of the rural communities in the West subject to impact.

Institutional Changes in the Community

The introduction of energy resource development stimulates a broad range of economic, political, and sociocultural changes in a small community. In the economic realm, occupational and wage structures change. New technical and skilled, high salary jobs are created while existing low salary positions in agriculture and service go unfilled. Because industrial work is organized around shifts rather than agricultural seasons, work in the community becomes more regimented (Denver Research Institute, 1979a). Not all citizens in the community can share in the new economic prosperity, however. Unskilled workers, the elderly, and women typically are not integrated into energy development.

Occupational life-style changes and population growth in the community also generate changes in social relationships. New roles are created, such as the position of city administrator or city planner in a community where formerly local government was administered by part-time elected officials. More positions are also created within existing roles. For example, more caseworkers are hired by the social services office or more neighbors are created as newcomers enter the community. Another change in social relationships occurs when old roles are redefined. Mental health professionals may find they are dealing with problems they have never encountered in the community before. A businessman's role changes as he is forced to respond to growth by seeking financing to renovate facilities and expand inventory. Finally, another extremely important role change occurs when individuals are replaced in existing roles. Those who have traditionally been in positions of power and influence may find their status in the community diminished: A county commissioner may be replaced by a younger or newer member of the community (Old West Regional Commission, 1975).

As social relationships change, new cultural issues and conflicts may also arise when various segments of the population express different traditions, values, and life-styles. One of the most serious boom town problems is conflict between the newcomers and long-term residents whose positions of power and authority and traditional life-styles are threatened by changes in the community.

Human Service Needs in the Energy-Impacted Community

With the rapid influx of population, human service needs become highly visible in the energy-impacted community. The sheer magnitude and suddenness of many institutional changes requires major adjustments by individuals. The requirement for rapid adjustment, in turn, generates increased stress, which may be manifested as human service needs in such areas as mental health, social services, health care, education, employment, youth services, and seniors' services.

With regard to mental health services, one of the problems that appears to predominate is an increased incidence of depression among women, due to such factors as isolation, lack of employment opportunities, and lack of support services (Moen and others, 1979; Holliday, 1979). Family crises also increase (Old West Regional Commission, 1979). Young adults newly arrived in the boom town face a number of mental health problems too by virtue of the fact that they have few solid interpersonal relationships, cannot easily become involved in recreational and social outlets within the community, and may be involved with drug and alcohol abuse (Uhlmann, 1978).

Children and adolescents are another segment of the population that is at risk in impacted communities. Youth are affected by such conditions as crowded living quarters, parents who are irritable as the result of long and/or odd-shift working hours, inadequate recreational facilities, and overcrowded schools that offer minimal programs (Gilmore and Duff, 1975; Uhlmann, 1978). Mental health and social service agencies report that juvenile caseloads increase dramatically. Child abuse cases, family problems, the incidence of runaways, and school problems demand more and more agency time (Old West Regional Commission, 1979). The demand for foster homes and temporary shelter for youth also increases, as well as the demand for daycare facilities (Uhlmann, 1978).

Although most information on mental health needs in boom towns is anecdotal, a current three-year longitudinal study of alcohol-related problems in energy-impacted communities is currently being conducted at the Denver Research Institute (1979b). To date, the findings indicate that per capita liquor sales increase dramatically during the boom period. In boom towns, as in other communities nationwide, alcoholism is more frequently a problem for males than for females. However, in boom communities the age of both males and females experiencing alcohol-related problems is much younger than national norms. In addition, newcomers have more problems than would be expected from their proportional representation in the community, although long-term residents are not without problems. For example, in one community researchers found that 36 percent of those seeking treatment for alcohol-related problems were newcomers, although they represented 12 percent of the population. Long-term residents constituted 64 percent of those seeking treatment; however, they comprised 88 percent of the community population (Denver Research Institute, 1979b, pp. 35–57).

Analysis of Increased Human Service Needs

One factor underlying increased human service needs in boom towns is the common disrupting experiences related to rapid growth: lack of adequate housing, inadequate community services and facilities, isolation for women and children, long working hours for men, and unfamiliar environments. The ordinary difficulties of relocation are compounded for newcomers in the community. For long-term residents, the community essentially becomes a new community because of the radical changes in the social, political, and economic structures (Cortese and Jones, 1977).

As a result of the changing composition of the local population, human service needs are also increased in the sense that new services are demanded. As young working-age adults and families with young children become proportionately larger groups in the community, special sets of needs that formerly did not exist must be addressed, such as day-care, family planning, and recreation services.

In addition to the disrupting experiences that lead to a rise in the incidence of human problems and the changing composition of the population, increased human service needs in boom communities are related to two other factors. The simple increase in the size of the population is one. The same problems arise in an impacted community as would arise in any community of comparable size. However, these problems are compounded, secondly, by the rate at which growth occurs.

To date research has not been conducted that would determine the relative magnitude of the effects of increase in scale as opposed to the effects of rate of change on increased human service needs. Several studies do suggest that human problems, such as child abuse, crime, or substance abuse, increase dramatically. For example, a study of Craig, Colorado (a community impacted by power plant construction and coal mining) reported a 623 percent increase in substance abuse, a 352 percent increase in family disturbance, and a 222 percent increase in crimes against property over a four-year period. During this time, the population of the county in which Craig is located grew by 47 percent (Lantz and McKeown, 1979). Similarly, reports on mental health admissions in Campbell County, Wyoming indicate that they increased 101.2 percent over a four-year period, while the population of the county increased 62.5 percent (Weisz, 1979).

Studies such as these do indicate that boom town growth produces social problems at a rate greater than population growth. However, the data are open to question on methodological grounds. If the Campbell County data are reanalyzed in terms of rates of admissions per thousand population, for example, quite a different picture emerges. This approach to analysis indicates that the rate per thousand has increased from .025 to .031 over the four-year period. Other methodological problems of studies of incidence include low reliability and validity of data because of variation in reporting and interpretation of data, lack of time series data, and wide variation in indicators chosen for analysis thus limiting the degree of comparability of data.

In conclusion, it is simply impossible on the basis of existing research to determine the exact magnitude of increased human service needs in relation to change in community size and rate of growth. Although there is no doubt that needs increase, most current information is anecdotal.

The Challenge to the Human Service Delivery System

Preimpact responses to human service needs in rural western communities included travelling long distances to obtain specialized services or meeting needs through family, friends, and neighbors. Such responses become increasingly unsatisfactory in a situation of rapid growth: The interpersonal networks that allow individuals to provide support to one another break down as radical changes in the physical and social environment take place. This breakdown of support systems affects newcomers and long-term residents alike. It has been analyzed as a process of urbanization that entails the loss and segmentation of personal relationships and their replacement by institutionalized services and impersonal and contractual relationships, as well as increased autonomy and anonymity (Cortese and Jones, 1977; Freudenburg, 1977; Gold, 1974).

Concomitant with the increase in human service needs and the diminution of interpersonal support networks in energy-impacted communities is an increase in the importance of human service delivery by institutions. In fact, the major changes in human service delivery that occur in boom towns are the location of new agencies in the community and an increase in the volume of services provided by existing agencies (Uhlmann, 1978). Unfortunately, the buildup of the service delivery system is usually slow, poorly planned, and inadequate to meet demand.

One of the major impediments to the expansion of the human service delivery system is the fact that in a rapid growth community the need for housing and municipal services is frequently given primary consideration, while the need for human services is neglected until problems reach crisis proportions. Human services are neglected by public officials and funding sources because they primarily require operating funds that are difficult to obtain, rather than capital facility funds, and because the results of investment in human services are difficult to evaluate.

Although timely provision of housing and municipal services does reduce human problems related to boom town growth, there are other factors to consider. Even when adequate housing and municipal services exist, other stresses of rapid growth accelerate problems. A survey in the boom town of Gillette, Wyoming, for example, indicates that respondents experienced moderate to high levels of life stress even though 75 percent were satisfied with their housing. Change alone, such as new employment or residence, generated stress (Weisz, 1979).

Lack of readily accessible money to support human services, as well as lack of professional manpower, are other impediments to the expansion of the delivery system. One of the hallmarks of an energy-impacted community is that the people and problems arrive several years before the tax base from the new industrial development is available to local government (Gilmore, 1976). Revenues available to the community in the initial stages of growth through taxes, bonding capacity, or reinvestment in the local community are low.

The major challenge to the human services system, then, is to provide adequate services in a situation of resource deficiency. Although energy-impacted communities have been faced with this challenge all along, the lack of resources available for human services is currently a national problem as a result of financial cutbacks engendered by such actions as the passage of Proposition 13 in California.

Our Response: The Wyoming Human Services Project

The Wyoming Human Services Project is a case example of an innovative response to human service needs in energy-impacted communities. It was originated in 1975 by a multidisciplinary faculty group at the University of Wyoming and was funded over a five-year period by the National Institute of Mental Health and other governmental and industrial sources. The basic plan of the program was to train students in professional curricula, such as social work, clinical psychology, nursing, law, recreation, or law enforcement to work as members of multidisciplinary human services teams. Once students graduated from the university, they were placed, on a yearly basis, in energy-impacted Wyoming communities.

In the community, team members spent one-half of their work time as professional staff members in human service agencies. In several cases, they undertook new roles within an agency or were involved in the initiation of a new agency in the community. The other half of the team members' time was spent working together on community human services projects, such as the establishment of a youth crisis home, a planned parenthood clinic, a drug and alcohol counseling service, a crisis line, or a discount plan for senior citizens.

The division of time between agency placement and community team-work was a crucial element in the program design. Agency experience acquainted the new professional with human service needs from the perspective of one segment of the community human service delivery system. When working on team projects, team members could then share their experiences with each other to arrive at a holistic view of the system. Using this perspective, the team then designed projects that would crosscut and coordinate the interests of a number of community agencies.

Although human service delivery is commonly organized categorically, there are a number of human service needs in a community that will not be addressed by this traditional service delivery strategy. These are the needs that are not primarily the responsibility of any one human service agency. For example, a caseworker in the social services office, a mental health clinician, and a police officer may all identify the need for a youth crisis program in the community; however, since their primary responsibility is to agency tasks, none would have time to devote to the organization of such a program. At the same time, the program would potentially benefit all.

It is the need for such programs and facilities that multidisciplinary human services teams can address. Such teams, with members freed from specific agency responsibilities, can accomplish the tasks that are necessary to establish a project or program that crosscuts agency interests. Since a multi-disciplinary team draws members from a variety of agency affiliations and professional backgrounds, it has the additional advantage of having a wide range of skills and knowledge available through its members.

Over the five-year life of the Wyoming Human Services Project, seven multidisciplinary teams have been placed in three rapidly growing Wyoming communities. Project evaluations have indicated that the program has been an extremely successful approach to meeting human service needs in energy-impacted communities. It provides a model of a workable response to scarce human and financial resources for human service delivery. Nationally, such integrating approaches to human services are also becoming increasingly common responses to diminished public support for human services (Gollub and others, 1980; Hagebak, 1979).

Conclusions

Prior to the 1970s, an exodus from rural communities in the United States occurred as the young migrated to urban areas in search of employment. Many of the current social problems and human service needs, such as erosion of the tax base available to support human services and deficiencies of professional manpower, have been related to and compounded by this basic demographic trend.

The post-1970 era, however, has brought a reversal in the out-migration trend (DeJong and Humphrey, 1976; Schwarzweller, 1979). Nationwide, rural areas are growing at higher rates than metropolitan areas. Factors influencing this growth include the location of services-related industries in rural areas, the development of recreational communities, the development of retirement communities, interstate highways that allow people to commute longer distances to work, and quality of life choices (Ploch, 1978; Wardwell, 1977). As a result, rural communities are likely to receive a sizeable population increase (Ploch, 1978). Although there are positive aspects to rural growth, there are also potential negative consequences, such as problems of social integration and fiscal deficits (Schwarzweller, 1979).

Rural, energy-impacted communities in the West are a special subset of rural communities and share some of the characteristics of other rural communities in the United States. Previously experiencing loss of population, they are now experiencing rapid population growth. Like other rural communities, their human service needs are great. As this article has shown, they too experience problems of social integration and fiscal deficits. Lessons learned about human service needs and delivery systems in the boom town may therefore be helpful in understanding the current general phenomenon of rural growth as it relates to human services issues.

References

Baumheier, E. C., Derr, J. M., and Gage, R. W. *Human Services in Rural America: An Assessment of Problems, Policies, and Research.* Denver: Center for Social Research and Development, University of Denver, 1973.

Cortese, C. F., and Jones, B. "The Sociological Analysis of Boom Towns." *Western Sociological Review*, 1977, *8*, 76–90.

DeJong, G. F., and Humphrey, C. R. "Selected Characteristics of Metropolitan to Nonmetropolitan Area Migrants: A Study of Population Redistribution in Pennsylvania." *Rural Sociology*, 1976, *41*, 526–538.

Denver Research Institute. *Socioeconomic Impacts of Western Energy Resource Development.* Denver: Industrial Economics Division, Denver Research Institute, University of Denver, 1979a.

Denver Research Institute. *Alcohol-Related Problems in Energy-Impacted Communities.* Denver: Social Systems Research and Evaluation Division, Denver Research Institute, University of Denver, 1979b.

Freudenburg, W. R. "Subjective Responses to an Energy Boom Town Situation." Paper presented at the 72nd annual meeting of the American Sociological Association, Chicago, Sept. 5, 1977.

Gilmore, J. S. "Boom Towns May Hinder Energy Resource Development." *Science*, 1976, *191*, 535–540.

Gilmore, J. S., and Duff, M. K. *Boom Town Growth Management: A Case Study of Rock Springs-Green River, Wyoming*. Boulder, Colo.: Westview Press, 1975.

Gold, R. L. *A Comparative Case Study of the Impact of Coal Development on the Way of Life of People in the Coal Areas of Eastern Montana and Northeastern Wyoming*. Missoula: Institute for Social Science Research, University of Montana, 1974.

Gollub, J. O., Henton, D. C., King, J. R., and Waldhern, S. A. *Rediscovering Governance: Using Nonservice Approaches to Address Social Welfare Problems*. Menlo Park, Calif.: Center for Urban and Regional Policy, SRI International, 1980.

Hagebak, B. R. "Local Human Service Delivery: The Integration Imperative." *Public Management Forum,* November/December 1979.

Holliday, G. "Effects of Energy Development on Rural Women." In *Energy Resource Development,* proceedings of a conference sponsored by the U.S. Commission on Civil Rights. Washington, D.C.: U.S. Government Printing Office, 1979.

Lantz, A. E., and McKeown, R. L. "Social/Psychological Problems of Women and Their Families Associated with Rapid Growth." In *Energy Resource Development,* proceedings of a conference sponsored by the U.S. Commission on Civil Rights. Washington, D.C.: U.S. Government Printing Office, 1979.

Moen, E., Boulding, E., Lillydahl, J., and Palm, R. *Women and Energy Development: Impact and Response*. Boulder, Colo.: Institute of Behavioral Science, 1979.

Old West Regional Commission. *Construction Worker Profile: Final Report*. Washington, D.C.: Old West Regional Commission, 1975.

Old West Regional Commission. *Socioeconomic Longitudinal Monitoring Project: Final Report*. Laramie: Center for Urban and Regional Analysis, Institute for Policy Research, University of Wyoming, 1979.

Ploch, L. A. "The Reversal in Migration Patterns—Some Rural Development Consequences." *Rural Sociology,* 1978, *43,* 293–303.

Schwarzweller, H. D. "Migration and the Changing Rural Scene." *Rural Sociology,* 1979, *44,* 7–23.

Uhlmann, J. M. *Providing Human Services in Energy-Impacted Communities*. Denver: Rocky Mountain Regional Office, Economic Development Administration, U.S. Department of Commerce, 1978.

U.S. Department of Housing and Urban Development. *Rapid Growth from Energy Projects: Ideas for State and Local Action*. Washington, D.C.: U.S. Government Printing Office, 1976.

U.S. Region VIII Department of Energy. *Regional Profile Energy-Impacted Communities*. Denver: Region VIII Department of Energy, 1979.

Wardwell, J. M. "Equilibrium and Change in Nonmetropolitan Growth." *Rural Sociology,* 1977, *42,* 156–179.

Weisz, R. "Stress and Mental Health in a Boom Town." In J. Davenport and J. Davenport (Eds.), *Boom Towns and Human Services*. Laramie: Department of Social Work, University of Wyoming, 1979.

Julie M. Uhlmann is a research anthropologist at the Denver Research Institute, University of Denver. She was formerly on the faculty of the University of Wyoming, where she was principal investigator and first project director of the Wyoming Human Services Project.

The Veterans Health Care Amendment Act of 1979 (PL–96–22) spawned the rapid development of a new program by the Veterans' Administration. Nationwide, about ninety Vet Center Programs are delivering service to the estimated 20 to 50 percent of Vietnam veterans who are continuing to suffer symptoms of post-traumatic stress disorder. Development of this public health service in Appalachia presents many challenges: A high proportion of combat veterans are concentrated in rural areas where traditional mental health services are limited.

Appalachia's "Forgotten Warriors": Outreach Services for Vietnam Veterans

Steven Giles

By the war's end in 1973, nearly three million American men and women had served a tour of duty in Southeast Asia. In the war, 57,000 Americans were killed and over 300,000 wounded.

Research on the survivors of the war suggests that 20 percent of those who served in Southeast Asia are still suffering from readjustment problems. A recent study by Wilson (1980) gives evidence suggesting that as many as 60 percent of the veterans who saw combat are continuing to manifest symptoms related to their war experience.

With the development of the third edition of the Diagnostic and Statistical Manual (DSM-III) the problem has been designated an official title. The diagnosis is post-traumatic stress disorder. In the case of the Vietnam veteran, it is often referred to as delayed stress, post-Vietnam Syndrome or simply PVS. The syndrome is characterized by a predictable response to having experienced a traumatic, usually life-threatening event. In Vietnam veterans, this means a reexperiencing of the trauma through dreaming or flashbacks, a numbing of affective responsiveness to the world, chronic low-grade arousal, feelings of estrangement, and guilt about survival or actions that were required in order to survive.

For at least 600,000 soldiers, the war is still not over. For this group, time has not been a sufficient healer. Their problems are actually intensifying as they reach mid-life. This represents a public health problem of major proportions.

Veterans' Administration's Operation Outreach

For years, Vietnam Veterans' activist groups have advocated that the Veterans' Administration (VA) recognize the prevalence of the problems experienced by those who participated in the Vietnam War. They have demanded that the VA develop programs that would provide help for the veterans who are still troubled by emotional, vocational, medical, and educational problems.

With the Carter appointment of Max Cleland as Administrator of Veterans' Affairs, the Vietnam veteran suddenly had a strong advocate at the head of the VA. Cleland is himself a disabled Vietnam veteran. It has been his highest priority to develop the necessary programming.

The cornerstone of this programming is Operation Outreach. This is a rapidly implemented program consisting of the development of approximately ninety Vet Center programs on a nationwide basis. Each state has at least one Vet Center. The programs are staffed with four members, including support staff. The staff is generally composed of psychologists, social workers, and paraprofessionals. The centers are in storefront locations with an emphasis on active casefinding, an informal and personal approach to the veteran, and an emphasis on involvement with the veteran's family.

Centers are expected to develop services addressing the particular needs of the veterans in their geographic area. Programs are expected to be modified to address the cultural context of the veteran population being served.

The Outreach effort is designed to reach the many veterans who have not taken advantage of the medical, mental health, vocational, and educational benefits available to them through the VA. In addition to outreach, the teams are providing direct service through individual and marital counseling. There is a strong emphasis on "rap groups" as a therapeutic method of dealing with the isolation and blocked affect of the veterans. Finally, teams are expected to develop a network of community-based referrals and to provide consultation and educational services to organizations to enhance their ability to relate to the problems of the Vietnam veteran.

Two other developments within the VA have been designed to address the particular problems of the Vietnam veterans. In April 1980, the VA officially began to recognize the constellation of symptoms experienced by many of the Vietnam veterans as a compensatable disability. By the summer of 1981, the VA will have developed a fee basis program that will allow in certain situations (such as isolation from an available Vet Center) community mental health providers to be reimbursed for care of Vietnam veterans referred to them by the Vet Center.

Appalachian Vietnam Veterans

As Operation Outreach continued its rapid development, it became clear that upper level administrators were insensitive to the issues of mental health service development in rural areas. Because urban minority group veterans were identified as a primary target population, all Vet Center programs were placed in metropolitan areas. Teams in rural states were placed in the largest city available and encouraged throughout training to aim their service at minority group populations.

Although the problems of urban veterans are undeniable, there is a programmatic underemphasis on the problems and needs of rural veterans. While, overall, states contributed rather evenly to military service during the Vietnam era (approximately 40 per 1,000 population), dramatic trends appear when the rates of those in service are compared to those who were actually sent to Southeast Asia. Fifty percent of rural military men were sent to Southeast Asia as compared to only 25 percent of urban military men. These figures are based on comparisons of twelve rural states—South Dakota, New Mexico, Idaho, North Dakota, Iowa, Montana, Maine, West Virginia, Mississippi, Vermont, Wyoming, Arkansas (those with over 60 percent of their population in nonmetropolitan areas)—to twelve urban states—Ohio, Florida, Michigan, Pennsylvania, Illinois, New York, Maryland, California, Rhode Island, Massachusetts, Connecticut, New Jersey (those with over 80 percent of their population in metropolitan areas). The rural rates for those who went to Vietnam ranged from 36 percent for Arkansas to 75 percent in South Dakota. The urban rates ranged from 16 percent for Maryland to 33 percent for Florida.

Casualty rates support the contention that rural men were the majority of those selected for combat roles. The five states with the highest casualty rates in the Vietnam War were West Virginia (39.9 deaths per 100,000 population), Oklahoma (36.6), New Mexico (36.5), Montana (35.2), and Alabama (33.6). The five states with the lowest casualty rates were Connecticut (18.9), New Jersey (19.4), Delaware (21.2), Vermont (21.2), and New York (21.8). Rates for the twelve rural states described above were 50 percent higher than those of the urban states (Veterans' Administration, 1979).

Socioeconomic and cultural influences are responsible for the Appalachian overrepresentation in combat roles. On the economic level, the draft affected the region's population disproportionately. The military draft has always drawn heavily from the groups that make up much of Appalachia's population—the working class and poor. Deferments from the draft to pursue an education, an option for many young men during the early years of the Vietnam War, were not viable for most Appalachians.

Appalachia continues to be characterized by tremendous poverty and limited vocational opportunities. Coal mining, which is often the only employment available, is in many ways as dangerous as combat. For many Appalachians, the promise of a steady income and vocational training offered by the military becomes a serious option in an area of severely limited opportunities.

In addition, many cultural factors make Appalachians good candidates for combat. Appalachia was originally settled by soldiers and other settlers who were willing to struggle to survive in the mountains. O. Normal Simpkins (1977) points out that many families received land in Appalachia as reimbursement for fighting in the Revolutionary War. It was a kind of G.I. Bill of the late eighteenth century.

Specifically, Appalachian males are hunters. At a very early age, they received training in the use of weapons, woodsmanship, and tolerance of the physical discomfort that accompanies hunting. This early experience is good training for the combat soldier. It is more efficient to select these pretrained men than it is to train an urbanite in how to survive outdoors and how to shoot a weapon straight.

Appalachians have always revered their soldiers. Most went to war for their country without asking questions. Appalachian soldiers performed well in combat. Traditionally, they did not defy authority. Their lives often included exposure to and tolerance of violence. Appalachians have always been people of action as opposed to contemplation.

Program Development

The development of a public health oriented service for Vietnam veterans of the Appalachian Region must address the accessibility of the target population to the service being offered and, more importantly, the acceptability of the service to the Vietnam veterans. Two critical sets of factors related to acceptability that affect the delivery and utilization of mental health services in rural areas have been identified by Wagenfeld (1977). The first set of factors is those values held by the client or the social structure in which the client lives; the second is those qualities inherent in the nature of the service provided.

Appalachian Values. In Appalachia, there are many commonly held values that must be considered when health care services are developed. Weller (1965) has pointed out that mountain people have strong negative attitudes about people who work in the helping professions. He further states that Appalachians are afraid of illness and that they delay getting care for fear that something may be wrong with them. "What is said about sickness in general is all the truer for mental illness; the mountaineer cannot accept it. 'Poor nerves' or 'worn out nerves' can be blamed for such disturbances. The psychiatrist's cure can be accepted only if he is called a 'nerve doctor.' The whole subject of mental illness is simply foreign to mountain people" (p. 119).

Another cultural variable that affects service development is the Appalachian intolerance of bureaucracies. Appalachians emphasize personal and face-to-face relationships and are confused by the impersonal structure of bureaucracies. The Appalachian fears those health care providers who use complicated language, rigid time schedules, and uncertain explanations.

In *Everything in Its Path,* an excellent study on the effects of the Buffalo Creek flood, which killed 125 West Virginians and destroyed their community in February 1972, Kai Erickson (1976) describes many of the values that influence Appalachians' reaction to stress and responsiveness to help.

A primary coping strategy of Appalachians, according to Erickson, is a pervasive fatalism. Other experts on this region have observed the same characteristic. Weller (1965) writes: "The sense of fatalism that runs through all of life comes into prominent play in medicine . . . . (It provides) a cushion for the mountaineer's heart against the rough times of his life — the death of the children, the killing of the husbands in the mines or woods" (p. 120). And war.

This passivity in the face of misfortune or sense of resignation is a cultural adaption to the physical and economic hardships of the region and the lack of control over events. The numbing caused by exposure to trauma in Vietnam does not often generate a great deal of concern in Appalachia. It is often labeled as bad nerves and may only become a treatment concern when the symptoms become very severe.

Bad nerves is rapidly becoming a prevalent, culturally accepted form of self-diagnosis for certain disabling conditions. It is basically a medical model or somatic notion that something is physically malfunctioning.

According to Erickson (1976) "the fear of disability has become a prominent theme in (Appalachian) thinking" (p. 87). He suggests that because of their history of physical sturdiness and survival ability, Appalachians have been preoccupied by physical health. Like others who share this concern (athletes, dancers, beauty contestants), their major apprehension is about their health, and they are consumed with concerns about their aches and pains.

Regional values must be carefully examined during the planning stage of any new human service program. This is particularly true in Appalachia, where a long history of inadequate health care resources have added to the problems of acceptability.

Service Barriers. The treatment of mental illness has intrinsic qualities that serve as barriers to service delivery and acceptance. This is particularly true in Appalachia. The modalities of mental health treatment have generally been developed by upper middle class therapists and researchers to be used on upper middle class clientele. It could be said that the treatments are most effective for those who need them least. Schofield (1964), in his critical review of psychotherapy, maintains that the best candidates for psychotherapeutic treatment are young, attractive, verbal, intelligent, and successful.

This is sometimes referred to as the YAVIS Syndrome. These adjectives are not often used to describe the people of Appalachia.

Appalachians are particularly sensitive to "foreigners" (anyone from outside the region) and have difficulty accepting help from anyone not in their reference group. Mental health professionals in Appalachia tend to come from other parts of the country and are generally from middle-class backgrounds. Many of West Virginia's physicians are foreign born. It is not unusual to hear Appalachians bemoan their inability to understand the language of their physician.

Also intrinsic to mental health care is the stigma that is attached to receiving care. Bentz and his colleagues (1971) have found that in rural areas the stigma associated with treatment is particularly intense.

The West Virginia Vet Center

As the first months of development and implementation are completed, the West Virginia Vet Center has successfully consolidated a position in the Huntington area.

Indigenous staff with the necessary professional credentials were hired. This was possible in an area without enough professionals only because federal salaries were higher than those paid by surrounding community agencies. The paraprofessional staff members were attracted because of their personal commitment as Vietnam Veterans to assist others in the "brotherhood." Having their roots in the region, the Vet Center staff members are sensitive to its culture. As a result, there is a reduced resistance by Vietnam Veterans to seeing the center as a useful program.

A major focus is total team involvement. The team secretary, who has first contact with many veterans, is a skilled paraprofessional who is a part of the treatment program. These initial contacts are a crucial phase of providing complete service.

The initial months of Vet Center activity were spent in community education, needs assessment, and the logistics of choosing and developing a site. The Vet Center staff encouraged local Vietnam veterans to meet to discuss concerns about the program and give advice on what needed to be offered.

Since the Vet Center is a VA program, many veterans have remained skeptical of the program's sincerity, capabilities, and credibility. Discussion of these concerns is always encouraged. Weekly meetings continue with a group numbering from three to ten veterans. The group is now attempting to organize as an independent Vietnam veterans advocacy group, which is sorely needed in the community.

Out of these meetings came a challenge that the team accepted and that has served as the nucleus of team development and credibility. Specifically, the team was asked to serve as advocate for a local Vietnam veteran who was incarcerated pending trail for holding a church congregation hostage. Holding the congregation hostage was his method of dramatizing grievances regarding the plight of the Vietnam veteran and his personal frustrations with the system. His behavior clearly stemmed from post-traumatic stress disorder. The Vet Center's involvement may help make a difference between his being incarcerated as a criminal or being treated. While not yet resolved, this case has become symbolic of the Vet Center's new presence in the community.

A great deal of effort had to be put forward to justify our program within the VA system. During a period of fiscal belt tightening, Operation Outreach was dubbed a pet project of Cleland's. Many resented that programs were being cut to accommodate the new Vet Centers. A great deal of extra energy was required by VA personnel to implement the program rapidly in a system lacking a reputation for speed.

To survive these kinds of pressures, the developing Vet Center staff spent many hours in the VA facilities. In-service education about the needs of Vietnam veterans was held with medical care and veterans' benefits services, and the strategy appears to have been successful. The program has developed links with community and VA agencies.

During the four-month implementation phase, approximately 100 veterans had direct contact with the Vet Center. The majority had been involved in heavy combat. As was anticipated, they were skeptical, angry, and had major difficulties with jobs and personal adjustment to civilian life. In particular, the majority of these men had recently experienced problems in their marriages.

Outreach service, rap groups, individual and marital counseling have all been established. Community education projects have been implemented and well received. The two community in-service programs given to date attracted an average of thirty-five participants each from community agencies. A recent open house attracted eighty-five guests. Community interest in the program continues to be high.

Community education focuses on a reduction of the sense of stigma associated with mental disability. Psychiatric jargon is avoided. Post-traumatic stress disorder is described as a natural consequence of exposure to life-threatening situations. Vietnam veterans are told they are not crazy but rather survivors. Television, radio, and the news media have all been very responsive to the program's presence in the community and have treated the center very well in both news and feature presentations.

The program is developing an approachable, informal atmosphere. The national Vet Center motto is *Help Without Hassles*. There is very little bureaucratic feel to the program. The veterans involved to this point often remark about the accessibility, the lack of paperwork, and the emphasis on action. The introduction of an ombudsman into the VA system has brought quick results in many cases and has helped program credibility. The service provided always addresses the veteran's own definition of the problem. No pressure is used to encourage treatment involvement or continued contact. First names of clients and staff members are used. Dress is informal.

The Vet Center is a drop-in as well as scheduled appointment service. The coffee pot is always full. This atmosphere appears to address the regional cultural values of personal orientation, loose time structure, and intolerance of bureaucracies.

The Outreach effort is focused on geographic extension. Although the staff is small, two itinerant staff members are available in areas of high veteran concentration. This increased accessibility is necessary in an area of minimal public transportation where poverty makes mobility impossible.

The only failure, to date, has been the center's inability to undo the deep distrust of institutions. The Vet Center is affiliated with the VA, which is perceived as part of the government. Added to this cultural response is the additional mistrust many veterans have of the VA as a result of not discriminating between the VA and the military, a history of unsatisfactory service from VA programs, and so forth. Once veterans get involved in the program, they stay involved. Getting them to come for the first visit, however, has been difficult.

Treatment Issue

In the cases where counseling becomes necessary, a major emphasis is placed on structure and education. Veterans are told what to expect from counseling and how it works. Those who have already been involved are used to educate new veterans to the helping process. The rap groups have been successful in achieving the continued participation of those who join them. Veterans are talking about their experiences for the first time and getting the kind of peer support needed to express themselves. The usefulness of psychotherapeutic techniques with Appalachians is supported by this experience.

The case should remain open regarding the effectiveness of traditional psychotherapy for Appalachians. A therapeutic alliance in Applachia requires personal concrete language and education about the treatment process. The Appalachian has personal resources to bring to bear on emotional problems. Recognizing the problem as one of the "nerves" means recognizing the source of the problem as internal. Appalachians are patient, far more than most mental health professionals are.

The challenge that remains is for rural mental health providers to avoid imposing their middle-class values on people they are trying to serve. Those interested in working clinically with rural populations should examine their motives and attitudes very carefully. A personal counseling experience might be useful for those considering working in rural areas. Also, it is quite necessary to rid oneself of romantic notions of rural America. It is all too easy to become frightened of poverty and personal suffering. Appalachia has more than its share.

References

Bentz, W. K., Hollister, W. G., and Edgerton, J. W. "Assessing the Stigma of Mental Illness." *The Psychiatric Forum,* Winter 1971, 17–22.

Erickson, K. *Everything in Its Path.* New York: Simon & Schuster, 1976.

Figley, C. R. *Stress Disorders Among Vietnam Veterans.* New York: Brunner/Mazel, 1978.

Schofield, W. *Psychotherapy: The Purchase of Friendship.* Englewood Cliffs, N.J.: Prentice-Hall, 1964.

Simpkins, O. N. "Culture." *Mountain Heritage,* 1977, *3,* 24–42.

Veterans' Administration. *Data on Vietnam Era Veterans: September, 1979.* Washington, D.C.: Reports and Statistics Service, Veterans' Administration, 1979.

Wagenfeld, M. O. "Cultural Barriers to the Delivery of Mental Health Services in Rural Areas: A Conceptual Overview." Address presented at Conferences on Rural Community Mental Health, Rockville, Maryland, May 5, 1977.

Weller, J. E. *Yesterday's People: Life in Contemporary Appalachia.* Lexington: University of Kentucky Press, 1965.

Wilson, J. P. "Toward an Understanding of Post-Traumatic Stress Disorders Among Vietnam Veterans." Testimony before U.S. Senate Committee on Veterans' Affairs, Washington, D.C.: May 21, 1980.

Steven Giles is a clinical psychologist and team leader of the West Virginia Vet Center. He has recently been involved in research on the epidemiology of mental illness in Appalachia.

Deinstitutionalization is a misnomer. An institution is a social organization that has continuity through time and is not dependent on the efforts of a single individual. The question is not one of institution versus no institution but rather small versus large and near versus far away.

Deinstitutionalization in a Rural State: The Vermont Experience

Hans R. Huessy

Deinstitutionalization, as applied to the treatment of the chronically mentally ill, has come to mean their removal from large, often antitherapeutic, mental hospitals to community settings. From a sociological point of view, however, this term is a misnomer: Patients are not being moved from an institution to no institution. Rather, there is a shift from large, distantly located institutions to smaller, more proximally located ones. In this sense, deinstitutionalization refers to the care of the mentally ill in smaller community settings. This chapter will consider deinstitutionalization in a rural state — Vermont — and will suggest some strategies for dealing with the problem in other areas.

The Historical Setting

Vermont and Wisconsin have probably had the most successful deinstitutionalization programs. Both states are primarily rural and this is a great help. Both are relatively small but especially Vermont (with only 440,000 inhabitants), making it possible for a central office to keep track of everything that is going on and for good central leadership to have an impact throughout the state. The rural setting has many advantages — more homes with extra rooms in them, the availability of the outdoors to a majority of the patients, less problems with zoning. In urban areas there is a tremendous amount of segregation by socioeconomic status, often forcing chronic care facilities to locate themselves in slum areas.

The groundwork for deinstitutionalization in Vermont was laid under the direction of Dr. Jonathan Leopold, and the major push of the program was carried out under Dr. Robert Okin while both were commissioners of Mental Health. Dr. Okin managed to persuade the governor that, in order to carry out deinstitutionalization, he needed to be allowed for a while to finance both the state hospital and adequate social support services in the community. He saw that, while chronic patients were being moved into the community, both the previous program and the new program must function simultaneously. In contrast, those states that were forced to reduce their hospital programs to make monies available for the community programs ended up with disabling inadequacies in both.

In the late 1950s Drs. Rupert Chittick and George Brooks of the Vermont State Hospital and Francis Irons, the director of the Vocational Rehabilitation Division for the State of Vermont, developed a rehabilitation program for chronic mental patients. Mr. Irons developed the concept of *training for living,* a pioneering venture adapting vocational rehabilitation methodology to the needs of chronic mental patients. Four halfway houses were set up, and the program was used as a model all over the world by the World Health Organization (Chittick and others, 1961). Now a twenty-year follow-up of the original cohort of patients is under way. Early in the program, patients taught us that the monitoring of medication and adequate social support were the essential ingredients for preventing rehospitalization. It was also documented that, for the chronic patient, immediate return to his or her own family carried with it a poor prognosis. Recently, Goldstein and Katon-Schwartz (1980) have replicated part of our findings, indicating that environmental stress and inadequate social support account for most readmissions.

A statewide community mental health clinic system was organized with the help of the original federal grants in 1948. By the time deinstitutionalization appeared on the horizon, there was a statewide network of locally run mental health services. An early after-care project was described along with many other Vermont mental health ventures in the book "Mental Health with Limited Resources" (Huessy, 1966). This original demonstration showed that a minimal after-care program could reduce rehospitalization dramatically. The program provided the monitoring of medication and minimal social support.

Spring Lake Ranch, founded in the early 1930s in central Vermont, is an example of an institution for the care of mental patients that effectively builds on its rural locale. One of the central tenets of the ranch is that, through family life and outdoor activity, chronic mental patients might find their way back to health. Over the years, the ranch has grown to have some fifteen buildings scattered over a hillside; it accommodates up to thirty guests, with a staff of about equal size (Huessy, 1966).

The hillside is accessible only by means of a steep dirt road that, at certain times of the year, is not passable except with special four-wheel-drive vehicles. The landscape, alternating between woods and open meadows, changes dramatically with the seasons.

This same landscape provides food, resources, work, and sport. In it a large vegetable garden flourishes; beef cattle and chickens live contented lives. The woods furnish maple sugar, lumber, and occasionally, venison; the lake gives an abundance of fish. Securing this bounty requires ample work, as do the necessary maintenance chores.

In addition, there is swimming, hiking, camping, skiing, and horseback riding. The efforts of many people have transformed a swamp into a tennis court, and recently a rustic gym was added to make a variety of indoor sports possible. At the bottom of the hill, a roadside store sells the products of the ranch.

Most guests need to develop a genuine independence, both in their work and from their families. Whereas the usual psychiatric institutions offer seclusion, the ranch offers geographical space and distance from family without the need for restriction.

Rural Vermont is ideal for the building of a small community such as the ranch, where ill individuals and their doctors can live together over long periods of time in an interdependent, close personal relationship, rather than in the often less dynamic, one-way professional relationship of doctor and patient current in many mental hospitals. From the beginning, a major goal of the ranch has been to simulate real life as closely as possible: There are no large, forbidding buildings; living is in small groups; staff and guests share accommodations. And, significantly, patients are called guests, and the doctors are lay persons called staff.

The rural world of Vermont structures life at the ranch, a life that responds to the seasons and virtually compels work. This work is one important element that saves the ranch from becoming just a caretaker. Work is a fundamental part of the program, not because it reflects the Protestant work ethic but because it gives individuals an opportunity to taste success, to feel useful, and more importantly, to build relationships with people when all else has failed. (Sweating together while digging a ditch can remove many a barrier!)

Because the work is necessary to survival rather than contrived for occupation, it gives meaning to the days. Whether it is planting and harvesting, clearing the winter roads, or cutting wood, the work is needed. Additionally in this rural setting, considerable labor that is required is of a simple nature, work that an unskilled person can perform and in the doing be successful.

Communal living and working combine to support the ranch's commitment to avoid the personal isolation observed in some institutions, an isolation that inhibits a patient's recovery by allowing him or her to retreat from the demands of the world. In a sheltered but unpaternalistic environment, the experiences on the ranch gradually equip and then compel a person to confront the world with confidence and a measure of independence. Communal living and working are combined with the most up-to-date pharmacotherapy (Wells, 1980).

Issues of Chronic Patient Care in Rural Areas

With increasing emphasis on the removal of chronic mental patients from large institutional settings, several related problems must be dealt with if the quality of their care is to improve: How their care is to be paid for; how caring itself is to be provided; and how the requirements of federal regulations are to be met. While these are generic concerns, they are especially relevant in rural areas.

It has been observed that, frequently, money is spent on certain services because they are reimbursable, not because they are necessary. The needs of mental patients can be divided into three areas: physical care, specific therapeutic interventions, and improving the quality of life. Reimbursement is generally available for the first two (even though the efficacy of specific therapies is often not demonstrated) but not for the third. Improving the quality of life is part of the process of caring—something that is not covered by third party payers. Caring is that special quality in human relationships that is not limited by work schedules and that goes beyond assigned tasks. It is what a mother provides for her children, and it cannot be bought from professionals. Our chronic patients no longer receive this caring from their own families. Caring for chronic patients is draining and exhausting, but it is essential for good patient care. The rural home operator provides family-type care for $356 a month. What he or she provides beyond the necessities of life is simply not financially rewarded.

By refusing to finance caring, third party payers continually push us toward greater professionalization. Professionals are needed to diagnose, to supply therapies as indicated, and to assess needs, but many of these needs must then be met by nonprofessionals. Not only can professionals not supply caring, they are further handicapped because patients tend to relate to them as substitute parents. Many chronic psychiatric patients have their most disturbed relationship problems with their parents. Such a patient can look upon nonprofessionals as peers and may be able to form successful relationships with them. For rural areas, with their chronic problems of manpower, the need for these caregivers is even more pressing.

How, then, does one provide this essential caring? Descriptions of the "burnout" of people working with adolescents or chronic patients are now common. We found ourselves dealing with this many years ago at Spring Lake Ranch and feel we have developed a model that could be applied to all programs involving the care of chronic patients. We began twenty years ago to recruit college students to come to work for one or two semesters. They came for minimal pay and devoted themselves intensely to our program while curtailing much of their personal life. We were gratified to see how these individuals could provide the caring we have just described. We now recruit a good part of our staff from young adults in or out of college who come for periods from three months to two years to supply this caring and in the process have a meaningful experience of self-discovery for themselves. Since their commitment is temporary, they can afford the limitations on their personal life that such work imposes. We do not train them in a formal way; they do not become therapists. They live with the guests, often as house parents, and share all other aspects of the work and social program with the guests. Our dream for the future is a national, voluntary service program that would supply a steady stream of people to work in institutions caring for chronic patients. Such a program could be built on the existing model of Vista and the Peace Corps. Not only could such a program provide the desperately needed caring for our chronic patients but it would also be excellent insurance against the deterioration of our many institutional settings. Because these individuals are not dependent on their superiors for their future careers, they feel free to speak up against any intolerable conditions without having to worry about the loss of their job. The steady stream of enthusiastic new individuals would also renew and invigorate our institutional settings and reduce the likelihood of their settling into a dull, institutional routine.

These young adults serve the important function of providing caring for chronic patients. Professional staff, however, are still needed to provide services for patients and their recruitment and retention in rural areas has been noted as a major problem (Cedar and Salasin, 1979). It is less of a problem in Vermont, as our state has become one of the most desirable locations in which to live. We have used outstanding consultants on an ongoing basis, if necessary flying them in weekly (Huessy, 1972). Such an approach can reduce professional isolation, improve the technical quality of the care provided, and furnish needed professional support to the staff. Ways must be found to use a small amount of very capable, professional help instead of depending exclusively on second- or third-rate professionals. This is particularly true for psychiatrists.

Finally, it has been frequently observed that one of the problems facing rural mental health relates to the inappropriate nature of federal regulations. Regulations governing mental health are most frequently promulgated in terms of an urban model of service delivery. (See the chapters in the present volume by Wagenfeld and Wagenfeld, Ozarin, and Blouke and Drachman for related points.) These are inappropriate in rural settings. Hodges, Fritz, and Fasso (1967) have made the point that federal regulations for community mental health programs often violate the notion of community. As an example, Vermont has recently been forced to join three truly separate, independent communities into one administrative unit because federal regulations on the population of catchment areas mandated it. Federal regulations whose benefits may, perhaps, have been established in an urban setting cannot be translated wholly to rural settings. To achieve optimum curing and caring for the patient, we cannot afford to be out of touch with the local community. We must respect the genuine community and work with it—often, despite regulations. It is only in this genuine community that one can hope to achieve integration of services. This notion of service integration is an important element of the Mental Health Systems Act now before the Congress.

References

Cedar, T., and Salasin, J. *Research Directions for Rural Mental Health*. McLean, Va.: The MITRE Corporation, 1979.

Chittick, R. A., Brooks, G. W., Irons, F. S., and Deane, W. N. *The Vermont Story: Rehabilitation of Chronic Schizophrenic Patients*. Burlington, Vt.: Queen City Printers, 1961.

Goldstein, J., and Katon-Schwartz, C. C. "Housing for Chronically Disabled Patients: Effect of Outcomes." Paper presented at 33rd meeting of the American Psychiatric Association, San Francisco, May 3–9, 1980.

Hodges, A., Fritz, K., and Fasso, T. "The Realities of Geographic Space in Rural Mental Health Programming." *Public Health Reports*, 1967, 5, 386–388.

Huessy, H. R. "Spring Lake Ranch—The Pioneer Halfway House." In H. R. Huessy (Ed.), *Mental Health with Limited Resources*. New York: Grune & Stratton, 1966.

Huessy, H. R. "Rural Models." In H. H. Barten and L. Bellak (Eds.), *Progress in Community Mental Health*. Vol. 2. New York: Grune & Stratton, 1972.

Wells, M. "Therapeutic Community Models: The Spring Lake Ranch." In E. Jansen (Ed.), *The Therapeutic Community*. London: Croom and Helm, 1980.

Hans R. Huessy was regional consultant in Mental Health for the Rocky Mountain Region from 1951 to 1953 and director of three county boards of mental health in northern New York State from 1953 to 1958. Dr. Huessy practiced community psychiatry privately from 1958 to 1964 and since 1964 has been on the faculty of the University of Vermont, Burlington.

A programmatic and fiscal interagency cooperative effort between the
Kennebec Valley Mental Health Center and Kennebec Valley Regional
Health Agency is discussed. This integrated approach to mental health
and medical services has reduced duplication of services and made optimal
use of funds in the Kennebec Valley area.

Integrating Mental and Medical Health Services: The Kennebec-Somerset Model

Carmen M. Celenza
David N. Fenton

Although Maine, with its multiple lakes and streams, rolling hills, and sparse population of one million people, enjoys the eviable reputation of being a vacationland, this same rural environment harbors a dearth of health services.

The Kennebec-Somerset area discussed in this chapter has a population of approximately 155,000 covering 4,900 square miles. The major population density of 130,000 people is concentrated within the Augusta-Water-ville-Skowhegan complex representing 1,700 square miles. In the northern region of Somerset County, with approximately 3,300 square miles, approximately 25,000 people are scattered among the various townships and plantations.

Public transportation within the Kennebec-Somerset region is virtually nonexistent; travel is primarily by private automobile, bicycle, or on foot. One train runs through the community on its way to Canada but makes no intermediate stops. In fair weather, it is possible to charter a plane to fly to the small landing strip close to the community of Jackman in the northernmost point of the area adjacent to the Canadian border. However, there is no scheduled air service to this community and surrounding area.

In the southern part of the Kennebec-Somerset region, where population concentrations are located, mental health and medical services have been adequately maintained. In the northern region, with its rural pockets, the delivery of medical and mental health services presents serious difficulties. While the medical community has made some inroads in this area, the provision of mental health services has been seriously lacking. There are a number of reasons for this deficiency, primarily the absence of adequate resources to deliver these services and the population's view that emotional problems are an abasement. The Kennebec Valley Mental Health Center has been concerned with this dearth of services and has initiated several attempts to resolve the problem.

The Center is a fully comprehensive community mental health center, governed by a board of directors and grounded in a community-based support system. With the passage of the Community Mental Health Centers Act of 1963, the Center received a staffing grant from the National Institute of Mental Health allowing it to expand both programs and geographic coverage.

Earlier Model

In 1975, the Mental Health Center agreed to take aggressive steps in addressing the needs of the rural area. A psychiatric social worker was hired with the specific understanding that he would live in the rural area and become an integral part of the community. An office was secured for him with easy accessibility to local residents. Recognizing that community education must necessarily precede direct services, the social worker was encouraged to participate in a number of formal and informal community-wide discussions regarding a wide range of mental health issues. When the community discovered his past employment as a volunteer fireman, the social worker was soon invited to join the local volunteer fire department, an invitation generally considered a major entree into the community's social scene. Although the social worker was encouraged to spend as much of his time as possible within the rural area, he nevertheless had back-up services readily available to him personally and to his clients.

After approximately one year of visibility and community education, the social worker was advised to begin increasing his direct service time. At this point, problems began to escalate. Although he attempted to control abuses of his available time, it was inevitable that "sidewalk consultations" would become more persistent and intense. These excessive demands, together with a blurring of community expectations, contributed to an early burnout. It was unclear to the community whether they were speaking to the psychiatric social worker as a friend and neighbor or as a clinician (see Mazer, 1976). After two and a half years, the clinician was removed from the area and the center was forced to reexamine its conceptual model and commitment to this service.

Planning Stages

Reexamination led the center to form a Rural Mental Health Planning Committee whose task was to explore with service providers, service agency resources, and clients, their perception of mental health needs and possible service delivery models. Through face-to-face contacts in most cases and letters in some instances, the center received input from rural health centers, the Department of Human Service field office, the area general hospital, school superintendents, school guidance counselors, youth service bureaus, state police, community action programs, Regional Health Planning Commissioners, area ministers, physicians, municipal officials, members of the Mental Health Center's Board of Directors residing in those areas, rural clients, and the Regional Health Agency, which coordinates the rural health centers of the region. This process was essential in assessing needs and allowing the community the necessary input into the program.

Based upon the input of all these individuals and organizations, the Rural Mental Health Planning Committee analyzed the data and drafted a preliminary Rural Mental Health Plan that was distributed to the participating agencies for reaction before the final implementation plan was developed.

In order to cover effectively the rural population and maximize coordination with existing facilities, rural office sites were established cooperatively with the Kennebec Valley Regional Health Agency and placed strategically within the Somerset County Region. This site distribution brought mental health services closer to the population pockets of the rural areas and paralleled the human service facilities available in those areas. The central office of the Mental Health Center, located in Waterville, is still available for referrals for mental health services that could not be provided in the rural site (such as inpatient, emergency, day hospital, and after-care services).

Regional Health Agency Planning

At the same time the Mental Health Center was going through its planning stages, a parallel effort was undertaken by the Regional Health Agency. Recognizing that approximately 65 percent of the clients coming to the health agency were suffering from related psychological problems, the Regional Health Agency focused on the possibility of providing outpatient mental health services through these various sites. Although the two executive directors met regularly to discuss a wide range of issues and problems, little focus was placed upon the long- and short-term ramifications of this dual planning effort.

Only after both agencies had completed their planning was it recognized that a fiscal and programmatic interagency cooperative network would reduce duplication of services, make optimal use of dollars, and ensure accountability. The end result made it clear that both organizations retain the appropriate professional staff and resources necessary to pursue an integration of health services. The Mental Health Center had the appropriate mental health professionals of various disciplines, together with appropriate linkages to psychiatric resources, while the Regional Health Agency retained medical personnel and a community acceptance of health services that would facilitate the entree of mental health. This broad-range planning eventually led to the integration of mental and medical services for the Kennebec Valley Area.

Responsibilities

To staff the rural mental health site, the center formed a team composed of psychologists, social workers, and a psychiatric consultant. At present, the Mental Health Center devotes eleven person days per week to six rural office sites, five of which are affiliated with the Regional Health Agency. In order to maintain personnel continuity at each site, the same individual is routinely assigned, with specialized personnel available for supplement coverage or consultation as service needs demand. Members of this team meet once weekly for treatment and program planning and coordination, peer review, and supervision at the center's central office. The rural team is coordinated by the director of Outpatient Services for the Northern Region (*outpatient* being used generically).

Clients are referred to the rural site mental health professional by family, health care providers, attorneys, schools, physicians, clergy, municipal officers, and others. On-site service includes assessment, evaluation, diagnosis, treatment, referral, and linkage, while consultation and education are available for professionals, schools, and communities. Emergencies are dealt with on-site and, when necessary, referral is made to the main office of the center and the Center Inpatient Unit.

All services are evaluated by the center's established procedures, which include outcome evaluations of symptomatology and role performance, as well as client reaction to services. In addition, the center seeks feedback from referral sources in the community regarding the quality and responsiveness of the rural mental health community services. Such evaluations are used for self-corrective modification and for all aspects of the rural mental health program.

The Kennebec Valley Regional Health Agency, partner to the Kennebec Valley Mental Health Center in this program, operates thirteen distinct health programs including the Rural Primary Care Health Center (RPCHC). The

RPCHC presently consists of five centers and provides comprehensive services to isolated communities in a four-county area of central Maine. These centers were initiated with the assistance of federal support under a mechanism known as Help To Underserved Rural Areas (HURA), a research and demonstration program designed to improve rural health care delivery methods.

The first of these centers began providing service in 1976, while the rest have been phased in on a schedule that opens one new center approximately every ten months. Of the five centers now in operation, one has two physicians, two have a physician and a physician assistant, and two have a physician assistant assisted by part-time physician support. Additionally, each site has an R.N./health educator and a receptionist/bookkeeper. Administrative support is provided on a shared basis from the central office of the Regional Health Agency. Each health center, however, has its own community-based board of directors responsible for policy making.

As communities have increased their use of these health centers, the physicians and physicians' assistants who staff them have found themselves with less time to attend to the psychological problems that often exacerbate medical problems. Such medical professionals frequently lack the expertise to deal with complex psychodynamics.

It was the field staff who transmitted these concerns to the Regional Health Agency administration. At first the agency considered employing a mental health professional of its own. Initial assessment suggested that through a combination of reimbursement, fees, and grant monies, a psychologist could be supported provided that he or she would travel back and forth among the various health centers in order to ensure the highest possible productivity level. But without other mental health professionals on the agency's staff, how could the agency have been assured that it was providing quality mental health care? How would it have provided continuity of care and psychological and psychiatric back-up services? And, finally, what long-range effects would this involvement have had on the existing mental health system of the region?

Conceptualization of the Policy

Before these questions could be answered, a model had to be created that would serve as the foundation upon which the integration could begin. This model emphasized a synergistic approach: The collective effort of the two agencies would have a greater effect than both acting independently. Synergism, as a working concept, has been a major tenet of the Regional Health Agency since 1973.

Sharing resources among the fourteen individual programs had become a well established process within the agency. Particularly in the Rural Health Center Program, the agency had experienced an increase in staff productivity and resource effectiveness due to the integration of the several categorical services provided in the health center service area. As the health centers emerged as multiservice centers providing a wide range of social/health programs, the population's use of such centers climbed considerably higher. The synergistic effect of integrating different categorical services had become well accepted. But despite this recognition, merging of services provided by other agencies had not been attempted primarily because the cost of interagency coordination seemed to be greater than the benefits that would be derived by the health agency patients.

Steps Leading to Integration

As an organization, the two major goals of the agency were to reduce duplication of resources and provide the highest quality level of care. With these two perspectives in mind, an analysis was carried out, showing that in the short run an independent agency effort could be carried out expeditiously. However, the long-term benefits were substantially limited, and it became clear that it would be more appropriate to negotiate with the local Mental Health Center the possibility of joining forces in providing mental health services in the rural center network.

The Regional Health Agency recognized that both agencies had substantial resources and that, by integrating its efforts, considerable benefits could be passed on to the health centers. Since financial resources were likely to decrease in the future, by sharing resources at this time, there would be potential for considerable savings that could later be reallocated to meet other community needs. In addition, showing political authorities that the two agencies could work cooperatively and share each other's resources effectively would improve their standing in the eyes of county commissioners, state legislators, and congressional delegations.

Finally, and of equal importance, was the desire to provide practitioners with a stimulating work environment that, in turn, would contribute toward greater effectiveness and satisfaction in carrying out services. The achievement of integration would, in addition, serve to facilitate recruitment and retention efforts.

Once the decision to integrate mental health and medical services was made and it was agreed that this approach could provide the most expeditious and cost effective method of delivering services, a total commitment to integration had to be made by the executive directors of both agencies. Without complete acceptance of this concept at the top, the efforts would, as likely as not, deteriorate. This collaboration was facilitated by a history of such efforts in the past.

Assumptions and Advantages

Several assumptions about integration were made by the two agencies. The first was that services could be provided with greater cost efficiency.

Allowing trained professionals to carry out the most appropriate activities would greatly enhance effectiveness of treatment and reduce cost of operations. It was also assumed that linkage would make available to the Regional Health Agency the Mental Health Center's existing supervisory structure and in turn the benefits of a continuing dialogue and consultation with other mental health professionals. This relationship would also obviate the need for the agency to reinvent the wheels of supervision, in-service training and education, and quality assurance. Because of the Mental Health Center's links with the state mental hospital and the general hospital's inpatient psychiatric unit, continuity in the referral process between the field worker and Mental Health Center and the rest of the mental health system would be considerably streamlined.

The potential for a two-way continuity of care would also become actualized under such an integration. The Mental Health Center could in the future refer its own clients to the health centers for outpatient after-care services as well as medical treatment.

Admission procedures could also be simplified and, in many cases, duplication avoided. Patient records would be combined and case conference procedures dramatically improved because of the combination of the two admission procedures and the record system.

Through integration, recruitment and retention of skilled health professionals could be facilitated and improved. Two of the major reasons physicians and mental health clinicians leave rural areas are the lack of professional support systems and the isolation of the communities. Clearly, this had been a major drawback in the Mental Health Center's earlier approach of assigning a lone clinician to a rural area. Providers generally enjoy the challenge offered by working with other professionals. Increasing the staff spectrum does much to stimulate and challenge each of the practitioners and improves the retention of essential providers.

Services in the first health center were initiated in January 1979, with services phased in at other health centers over the following six-month period. After twelve months, the physicians and physicians' assistants all responded enthusiastically to the mental health service and rated it among the most useful and beneficial to their practice of all the shared activities provided centrally by the parent agency. In particular, physicians and physician assistants appreciated the availability of consultants and the educational services provided to them through case conference procedures.

Since the first year of this integration is coming to an end at the present time, cost data and client census information are not yet available. With the exception of one health center, patient response has been quite high. In the last quarter period, four of the five centers reported that sixty-nine different patients made 118 visits to the center to receive mental health services from the itinerant psychologist. These figures do not include the number of service units provided in the health centers by the back-up child psychologist. Bearing in mind that the psychologist spends only one afternoon per week in each center, that the mental health practice has had only a year to grow, and that three of the five health centers have been in existence for only two years, it would appear that use of services thus far has been remarkable.

Our other expectations have also proved true. We did, in fact, experience increased use of health services as new people became patients of the health center because of the availability of mental health services. In four of the five health centers, physicians and physician assistants expressed the belief that their time was better utilized and that they were more effective in their treatment because the service of a psychologist was available to them. Although few mental health patients cared for in the health centers require more intensive treatment, those who did gained easier entry into other levels of Mental Health Center services.

Continuity of care was considered by all to be improved by the availability of localized treatment. The cost of providing treatment did not exceed the budgeted expenditure as originally envisioned. Income, unfortunately, lagged substantially because the expected revenues, and the write-off rate for mental health services far outpaced that for medical services. Likewise, availability of third party reimbursement was sharply reduced with only Medicaid generally available.

Transportation problems for clients were also diminished and in a time of escalating gasoline costs, availability of services locally was of great advantage to local community patients. The intellectual and professional stimulation that health center practitioners provided for one another was as expected: Each physician's assistant specifically mentioned this as an incentive to continuation of employment.

The Mental Health Center derived significant benefits through this integration through cost containment and the communities' acceptance of mental health as an added and viable dimension to health care. A major condition of the integration was for the center to use the agency's facilities rent-free, together with the agency's back-up clerical services. Professional isolation was significantly reduced, and there was an increase in the intellectual stimulation available to professionals. Easier entry of the mental health system into local communities and an accompanying increase in the use of a grossly underused service was also apparent. Mental health clients felt more comfortable in coming to a health center facility when they knew that the community would have no way of knowing if they were being seen by the physician or the psychologist.

Problems

While there have been decided advantages in this interagency cooperation, there have also been serious barriers to coordination. Such barriers are a source of serious fragmentation of services not just between the two agencies but throughout the entire human service network. Invariably, a funding problem in one agency will adversely effect the other and a "domino effect" soon occurs, with possible contamination of two services rather than one.

Categorical funding mechanisms that identify specific allocations rather than providing the greatest flexibility of bloc grant allocations have proven to be a problem. The nature of categorical funding tends to discourage integration of existing services at the local level. Categorical funding sources also generally prefer to make awards to programs serving large populations with large budgets. The effects in rural areas have been particularly harmful because the small population bases put rural communities at a distinct disadvantage in competing for categorical grants. In turn, this lack of success in the competition for funds results in the limited availability of services. It is ironic that, in circumstances of scarce resources, integration must often be put aside.

Another basic area hampering integrated services is the territorial imperative of distinct agencies. Organizations have a tendency to protect and defend the scope of their services and to resist erosion of their authority. The effects of organizational turf problems upon integration are substantial. Some of the issues that must be addressed are who people report to and to which organization they hold their loyalty, which organization receives primary visibility and credit, and how expenses are allocated and reimbursement is distributed. The concept of professional turf also has a tendency to discourage cooperation between disciplines.

The model described in this paper subscribes to a generalist orientation for psychological services. The clinical psychologist was the clinician of choice for the rural area because of his or her versatility in diagnosing and treating a wide range of psychological problems, because insurance and third party payors would reimburse the cost of his or her services, and because he or she would have greater credibility with the rural health physician and community at large.

The community's attitude toward mental health could also be a barrier to integration. Acceptance of mental health as a major health resource has lagged behind the acceptance of other health services. On several occasions, providers on the Community Health Center Boards have questioned the wisdom of integrating medical services with a separate and distinct service. These potential problems have to be faced if integration of mental health services in the rural areas is to become a reality. Some of the concerns have proven to be real, others imaginary.

In the early stages of the planning process, steps were taken to confront the problems that have been discussed here. Such steps included the center's staff participation with the Mental Health Center in the selection of mental health personnel for the health centers. This participation encouraged the physicians' investment in implementating the service. The schedule of the phase-in process was also a decision in which health center practitioners had a primary role. The medical staffs were also enlisted to take the primary role in persuading the Health Center Boards of the advantages of this new service. In four of the five centers, the Boards were receptive. The management staffs of the two organizations spent considerable time working out agreements on protocols, fee charges and collection mechanisms, and integration of record systems. These proved to be relatively straightforward tasks. Attending to these problems in the early stages greatly facilitated relations between the actors and substantially improved the climate for the initiation of these services.

In looking back at the integration of the two services, several resources seem to have been particularly advantageous to the two agencies. Because both agencies were already regional in nature, their management was familiar with working in a decentralized system. Regionalization of services requires consensus and community participation, as well as familiarity with the pluralistic process that, in turn, eases the integration problems of a multisite system.

Perhaps the major strength of the integrated model was in the ability of the two agencies to capitalize on this regionalized concept. Clearly, the trend in community thinking today is the retention of local control of monies, services, and decisions leading to those services. In communities where mental health is still a new and alien concept, local visibility of mental health services accompanied by the presence of the local governing boards who control those services tends to facilitate the acceptance of mental health as an integral part of the health care network. In each of the health agency sites, local residents had a specific role in planning and implementation of services as well as a continuing role in the maintenance of sites. In most of these locations, residents took it upon themselves to beautify the buildings and make them presentable to clients and to the community for their various open-house functions. This same project ownership led to an advocacy system for the programs. Soliciting of funds at the local level became a community project, and local citizens advocated the funding of the agency to local communities and county government. Local citizens also advocated the retention of mental health services as an integral part of the total health care.

Perhaps one of the more important advantages of a regionalized approach to health care is in the community's awareness of what its specific service needs are. Historically, the service needs of an area have been handled by the central office of an organization following a peripheral survey. In our instance, needs were determined at the local level and subsequently submitted to the central office of the agency for integration into its organizational plan.

Finally, there existed a significant commitment on the part of the entire management structure in both agencies. On numerous occasions supervisory personnel from the Mental Health Center visited the health centers to meet informally with the physicians and evaluate the progress and performance of their personnel. Problems expressed by the physician and psychologist were quickly corrected, improved procedures initiated efficiently, and follow-up on suggestions always effectively delivered.

The integration of separate services is generally not easy. At this site, the process went smoothly and the results promised significant benefit to the two agencies and the clients whom they serve. The actual investment was minimal in terms of dollars, staff time, and physical resources. The synergistic effect of that investment exceeded everyone's expectations. In this particular effort, however, there were a number of resources available to the participants that helped assure the project's success. Others contemplating such efforts would be wise to assess whether they, too, share at least some of the same resources. For community agencies faced with meeting the dilemma of increased demands for services and reduced funding, integration may offer new hope. The difficulties encountered by two separate organizations working together are considerable and patience is essential. The potential for improved accessibility and reduced unit costs more than equals such difficulties.

Reference

Mazer, M. *People and Predicaments*. Cambridge, Mass.: Harvard University Press, 1976.

Carmen M. Celenza is executive director of the Kennebec Valley Mental Health Center and currently completing his second year as president of the Maine Psychological Association.

David N. Fenton is executive director of the Kennebec Valley Regional Health Agency and chairman of the National Rural Primary Care Association.

*In order for community mental health programs to be effective, they must
come out of a broad base of community support and involvement.
The historical development.of such a base is described.*

Community Support and Involvement in a Rural Mental Health Center

Edwin Fair

The Catchment Area

To appreciate fully the community support behind the Bi-State Mental Health Foundation, a rural comprehensive mental health center, it is important to look at the nature of its seven-county catchment area. In addition, we will describe, on a chronological basis, the development of our interaction with the community. Our catchment area has a historical background that is one of the most colorful in the Southwest. Indians and cowhands, sturdy pioneers and twentieth century oilmen—all have left their mark. Their achievements have given a distinctive character to this section of Oklahoma and Kansas.

Shortly after the end of the Civil War and during the late 1880s, this section of the United States was traversed by cowtrails from Texas to the railheads in the cowtowns of Kansas. Oklahoma was not yet a state. It was known as Indian territory in 1889, when a five-county area in central Oklahoma was opened for settlement. On September 16, 1893, with Arkansas City, Kansas, as the chief point of departure, a shot was fired as a starting signal for the largest and most dramatic of all of the land runs in United States history. By nightfall, virtually all of the claims in a six million acre area had been staked by homesteaders. To this, an economy built largely on wheat farming and cattle raising, was added a faster paced oil industry that brought millions of dollars of new wealth and thousands of new people into the area.

When the Bi-State Mental Health Foundation was started in 1968, the total population of the seven counties was 194,975—from 8,140 people in Grant County to 51,042 in Kay County. Virtually all of the residents are white, with small numbers of blacks and Native Americans. The most densely populated county (Payne) is the site of Oklahoma State University. Although the catchment area is rural, there are major industries in some of the counties and the existence of the university and a major oil company research facility give the area a relatively high median level of education. Those areas that have subsisted wholly on farming and ranching have experienced population declines, while counties with industrial development have shown growth.

Historical Development of the Mental Health Program

Prior to the establishment of the Kay Guidance Clinic, the forerunner of the Bi-State Mental Health Foundation, no mental health services were available other than those provided by local family physicians. The nearest public mental hospital care for Cowley County, Kansas, residents was 150 miles away. For Oklahoma residents the closest state hospital was 80 miles away from any community, and one community had to transport its patients 180 miles. At the time our program was started, there was one private psychiatric hospital in the state of Oklahoma and none of the general hospitals admitted psychiatric patients. Happily, this trend has changed over the past twenty years and many of the general hospitals now admit psychiatric patients.

In 1954 the Women's Association of the First Presbyterian Church in Ponca City inaugurated a survey to determine the need for a child guidance center for the city. This survey, completed in 1956, indicated the need for such services. Meetings were held among the various groups within the community and approximately 400 citizens from all over the county drove sixteen miles to the county seat to meet with county commissioners. The courthouse was too small to hold this many people and they held a meeting on the lawn. With such a demonstration of widespread county interest, the county Excise Board agreed to appropriate up to $500,000 to start a child guidance center program, but the county commissioners and the Excise Board pointed out that the State Legislature would have to pass a law before money could lawfully be appropriated for such services.

The Kay County Association for Child Guidance was formed and, in 1957, a committee of representative citizens was appointed to recruit professional staff for a child guidance center. Even though they waged an enthusiastic and aggressive campaign, they were successful in attracting only two psychiatrists who manifested enough interest to have personal interviews. Finally, the committee went to the Menninger Foundation in Topeka, Kansas, where they approached me. I accepted the position and have been the psychiatrist director ever since. We have often been asked about recruitment of staff for a rural mental health program, and believe it is of prime importance for the director to be interested and involved in building a community program for mental health. The professional person and his or her spouse must be convinced that the site is attractive and offers opportunities for a professional career and the rearing of a family. Cultural and recreational facilities, city government, the strength of the churches and their programs, and the overall attitude of the community should be evaluated by potential staff, as well as community involvement, the support of informed citizenry, the existing mental health needs, and the positive climate for creating a community mental health program. The mental health professional's spouse must be receptive to living in a smaller city and interested in the development of a community approach to mental health. In our case, I am the son of a country doctor and have an orientation to rural America, particularly rural Oklahoma. I was reared in an atmosphere where medical services provided by a dedicated father in general practice made for a broad interest in community mental health services. Since I had been a thoracic surgeon for several years, I had friends among many of the doctors in the community, some of whom had been classmates at the University of Oklahoma School of Medicine. Because of my background, rapport was facilitated with the professionals and citizens within the community. These relationships were of key importance in the development of the existing program.

A key factor in the ability of a program to attract staff is the foundation's policy regarding private practice. Our professional staff has had the privilege of being involved in private practice and, in the twenty-two years since the beginning of Kay Guidance Clinic, there has never been an issue concerning exploitation of the tax-supported program for the benefit of private practice. Instead, we have been able to recruit well-trained people who have remained loyal to the tax-supported program and this has given a stability to the professional staff.

In January of 1958, a full-time psychiatric social worker was added to the staff. I was employed twenty-six hours per week, and the clinical psychologist, who also came from the Menninger Foundation, was employed thirty hours per week. Approximately one year prior to the time I came to the program, I altered my training program at the Menninger School of Psychiatry so that I would be more knowledgeable about and sensitive to the needs of a community and could develop community support. On the basis of this training, I concluded there must be a working relationship between the clinic and the schools, both public and parochial, the ministerial associations, the medical profession, the legal profession, and the business community. During the first year the program existed, the staff made 240 appearances before various groups in Kay County, Oklahoma: I alone made 186 presentations. These presentations were to civic organizations, PTA groups, school boards, professional educator groups—including elementary, secondary, and college teachers—ministerial associations, various church groups, the bar associations, various medical and paramedical groups, child study groups, and fraternal groups. All these appearances were in the interest of promoting mental health and public support for the local mental health clinic.

A working relationship was established with the schools after meeting with the school boards and school administrators. Ours was a completely new service, and the responses from the people in education varied from a denial that there was a need for such services to a request on the part of the classroom teachers for all the help they could get. Educators showed an increasing acceptance of these services, with resulting requests for in-service training of teachers and counselors, as well as clinical services for children who had a need.

In 1959, in response to strong representations, the Oklahoma State Legislature passed a law allocating $500,000 for child guidance center services. The Excise Board of Kay County then allocated $250,000 of county tax funds for the operation of the child guidance center. Our initial error was to locate a private practice and the tax-supported program in the same office. This created confusion and it became necessary to separate the two; new housing for the tax-supported program was sought. The members of the Board of Directors of the Kay Guidance Association corporation signed personal notes for the purchase of a concrete block building. With this vote of confidence and the ever increasing need for services, other community support followed. The local labor unions volunteered their services after hours and on Saturdays to renovate the building from an industrial site to professional offices to house the child guidance clinic. The building was dedicated at an open house ceremony with participation of the members of the Board of Directors and many citizens who manifested an increasing interest in the new program for mental health. In 1960, the mayor of Ponca City, where the outpatient facility was located, proclaimed the week of March 20-26 as Kay Guidance Clinic Week and urged that citizens become acquainted with the work, aims, and objects of the group and lend aid, assistance, and encouragement to the furtherance of its program.

As the community became better acquainted with the clinic, increasing requests for services were received. Clergymen requested a training program to improve their counseling skills. Increased requests came from elementary school principals for in-service education. The secondary school counselors met with me to improve their counseling skills. The Ponca City Board of Education, through the county medical society, asked the clinic to provide a program of sex education services to the schools. The county medical society specifically requested that this program be conducted by me personally as psychiatrist director of the guidance center. This request came prior to the time that sex education became an accepted activity in public schools, and we recognized the delicacy of the issue, despite the apparent need for such a program. We decided that our guidance clinic would come into a school system with sex education programs only on the invitation of the boards of education and the superintendents of the school systems. In addition, all audio-visual aids used would be available for viewing by the parents of the students. The sex education program would be voluntary; no student would be required to attend and none would be criticized for nonattendance. The discussions would be taped and available to parents who were interested in the content of the program. The program would also have the approval of the ministerial association, as well as the county medical society. These requirements still remain in effect, and over the years the program has been expanded to include children at elementary school level and their teachers.

The staff of the Kay Guidance Association encouraged a small association for the mentally retarded to form an acting Kay County Council for Retarded Children. This resulted ultimately in the construction of a $400,000 Opportunity Center for the education and training of the mentally retarded. The members of the guidance clinic staff and the Board of Directors of the Kay Guidance Association helped the Kay County Council for Retarded Children in establishing the Cherokee Strip Golf Classic, which provides financial support for the Opportunity Center and the council for the mentally retarded. The support of the Guidance Association has continued. I have assisted in establishing a foundation for continued support and serve as a member of the Board of Directors of this foundation. It is projected that the foundation will in time have enough money to carry out the program for retarded children on the basis of funds received through the golf classic, as well as donations. This goal is within reach. Although, initially, the Opportunity Center did not receive tax support from the State Department of Education, state funds have been available since properly trained teachers for the mentally retarded child have been employed.

By 1963, the Kay Guidance Clinic had grown to the extent that surrounding counties were requesting similar services. More services were requested than could be delivered in available staff time. Waiting lists for service developed. However, community support allowed program expansion. In 1964, a ceremony marked the burning of the mortgage of the building that had been purchased by the Board of Directors who signed personal notes; the United States Congress had passed the Comprehensive Community Mental Health Center Act of 1963, providing funds for construction of mental health centers, and, after much discussion, the Board accepted federal funds to expand services to schools. The staff of the clinic increased to fifteen members.

In 1965, when Congress passed the Amendments to the Comprehensive Community Mental Health Center Act, establishing funds for salaries of professional staff, the Board of Directors once again discussed the expansion of our program. Our building, which had been bought and paid for, was too small. It was sold and the clinic moved to a former motel building. The Board approved an application to establish a comprehensive community mental health center.

Representative citizens from six counties in north central Oklahoma and one county in south central Kansas met to formulate preliminary plans for formation of the Bi-State Mental Health Foundation. Meetings were held with the superintendent and the trustees of the Ponca City Hospital to plan a cooperative program for inpatient services. Prior to this time, some inpatient services were available but on a limited basis only. During the preceding two years, the seven-county area had sent 456 people to the state hospitals, where the admission rate was increasing at approximately 20 percent per year. With our limited staff, we had seen 624 people from the one county served by Kay Guidance Clinic in that two-year period of time. The surrounding counties were now asking for mental health services.

As we were contemplating an application for federal funds for a comprehensive community mental health center, it seemed reasonable to establish the inpatient service in Ponca City. The one hospital in the community was run by the Sisters of Saint Joseph. Although the hospital administrator, a layman, advised the sisters and the trustees against initiating inpatient psychiatric services, community support was mobilized, as well as that of the medical community, which voted unanimously to advise the sisters and the trustees to establish an inpatient unit. The community even sent a committee to discuss this need to Wichita, Kansas, home of the motherhouse of the order. The sisters agreed to provide inpatient services as a part of the application for the comprehensive community mental health center. In the years that followed, they have been most supportive in providing such services. Although operating with limited tax money, the Sisters of Saint Joseph have continued to be totally cooperative. A patient has never been denied admission to the psychiatric service for any reason other than that all beds were filled.

In 1967, the Bi-State Mental Health Foundation submitted an application for a comprehensive community mental health center. A thirty-member Board of Directors was formed, with only one person declining the invitation to join. Repeated meetings were held in each of the counties. The president of Oklahoma State University became the first president of the Bi-State Mental Health Foundation. An adequate representation of physicians served on the Board to foster continued interest.

With the establishment of the comprehensive community mental health center, a wide range of services was added, including clinical pastoral services, departments of psychology, social work, speech, hearing, and education. The staff increased to eighty.

In fulfilling the requirements of federal legislation, additional programs were established, including one for the Native American community, the White Eagle Community Development Association, aimed at helping American Indian adults develop personal fulfillment. We also established pre-school programs and a halfway house for alcoholics. We started the 55 and Older Club, in order to help senior citizens socialize. An inpatient unit of twenty beds was established at the Sisters of Saint Joseph Hospital in Ponca City and two psychiatrists were added to the staff.

Satellite units began operating on the campuses of Oklahoma State University and Northern Oklahoma College and in Arkansas City, Kansas and Winfield, Kansas, with the central office and the outpatient department remaining in Ponca City.

Over the next ten years, community involvement and support continued to expand. The staff was influential in helping to form an interagency board of social services, a cooperative effort among the various groups in the community providing human services. The foundation helped develop a curriculum for use in the school system, kindergarten through twelfth grade, on drug abuse and drug education. The staff held seminars on these subjects. The Department of Education of the Bi-State Mental Health Foundation, in cooperation with the local television station, developed for the Ponca City Schools a series of TV training aids to help teachers in the instruction of children with learning disabilities. A pilot program in learning disabilities called "Special Training for Exceptional Persons" was conducted by the staff.

As our progam grew, it attracted attention outside our area. The *Daily Oklahoman,* the largest newspaper in Oklahoma, in a featured article, described the Bi-State Mental Health Foundation and its expanding program. An eleven-week summer course in clinical pastoral education was offered by the Department of Pastoral Care. In 1974, a federal grant was received for the expansion of children's services under our child development program. This was designed primarily to meet the needs of children from preschool years through the sixth grade.

By this time, the staff had outgrown the old motel building and the Board of Education of Ponca City leased us an older school building for $1.00 per year. This was a way of showing their appreciation for our work with the school system and our contributions to the community. This building has become the outpatient clinic and the administrative offices of the Bi-State Mental Health Foundation. The building was renovated and, although there are over thirty offices, it is still not large enough.

Other activities include psychiatric evaluation for the police departments of Ponca City, and Arkansas City, Kansas, of all police officers who are hired. In Cowley County we assisted the community in establishing a workshop program for mentally retarded and emotionally disturbed adults who needed a day hospital program: Participants in this program are evaluated in our mental health center. In Cowley County, we helped establish a home for boys who have come into conflict with legal authorities. The boys are evaluated in our mental health center and our professional staff serve as consultants on a regular basis to the house parents. One of the members of our staff also serves on their Board of Directors.

When Public Law 94–142, which relates to the education of the handicapped, came into existence, we met with school superintendents in our catchment area. We offered our services in helping establish a program for the emotionally disturbed, the child with learning disabilities, and the mentally retarded as they come into contact with the school system. Our association with the schools in this program depends entirely upon the needs and preferences of the school administrations.

Kansas now has legislation making local monies available for chemical abuse programs primarily in the area of alcohol abuse, and we are establishing a new program. This program involves a cooperative effort between the local municipalities, the county government, the school systems, and our community mental health centers.

What Has Experience Taught Us?

We have listed in a general chronological order the development of our program and our involvement in the community. Each program has required planning and implementation. We have had to learn to be aggressive, as we were in helping establish a program for the mentally retarded. We have also had to learn to wait, as we have done in working with the school systems. Experience has taught us that unless we have the support of a school superintendent who, in turn, will influence the Board of Education, we will not have an effective program in a given school system. If we have the support of the school administration, then we need the support of the principal of a given school. When we have that support, we become involved in a meaningful, working relationship with the classroom teacher. Although it is classroom teachers, essentially, who request our services, we sometimes have to wait until all the people involved are ready for services.

We have also learned that we can suggest a program or an idea and stimulate an interest while others in the community are given the privilege of developing the actual program. Our Help Line Program in Ponca City is a good example of this process. The program is a service available to people in the community who are in stressful situations or simply want to talk over their problems with someone on the telephone. The program has one paid employee, the other employees being volunteers who are trained by the staff of the foundation. An arrangement has been made with Northern Oklahoma College to provide college credit for the classes that the volunteers attend in preparing to be listeners in the Help Line Program. We were aware of the need of a program of this type and discussed it with one or two community-minded individuals, then waited for it to unfold in the community. Since the listeners must have training and since this training is provided by us, the community is aware of this ancillary service and, while it is not seen as one of our specific programs, it is recognized that the program could not exist without our support.

We are now helping to develop a program described as Parents in Crisis. Parents who are in need of services are in the process of establishing a community-wide group that will provide assistance in times of crisis. Various community service organizations are involved, along with the foundation. In all probability, in the not too distant future, we will be actively involved in counseling, educational, and therapeutic efforts with the various participants in this group.

Conclusion

Frequently we have visitors who inquire about our community involvement. The most common question asked is, "How did this all come to pass?" We are convinced that a program like ours must have the leadership of people who are oriented toward the community and see the importance of community involvement. Such leaders will set the pattern. If the director of such a program has this orientation, he or she is more likely to recruit staff members with similar outlook. In our case, one of the questions we ask of professional people who are added to our staff is how great an interest they have in community involvement. In a rural community, more than in an urban one, the staff members will present a positive or negative image depending upon their orientation, their skills, and their ability to relate to the citizens in the community under a variety of circumstances. They must be willing to be involved in the community outside of their professional relationship to it.

A danger to be guarded against is overextending services. We believe it is important for the staff to realize that each member has a valuable role to play in the delivery of services and each is important in the total program. The leadership in such a program needs to be aware of professional competition, of jealousies that may arise, and see that these are properly handled before they undermine staff morale. It is also important to share knowledge and skills. Otherwise, the individual in a rural community can feel professionally isolated. Proper opportunities for professional growth must be provided, and staff members should be encouraged to use them. The professional staff should serve as an advisory committee to the director and the Board of Directors. This committee needs to be functional and their recommendations given proper consideration. Staff members have a continued public relations role, one that need not be threatening and one that, after a while, becomes an automatic part of the operation of the program. In a rural area, this public relations role is very evident and not at all restrictive or uncomfortable.

Edwin Fair has been psychiatrist director of the Bi-State Mental Health Foundation in Ponca City, Oklahoma, since its inception.

An effective educational program needs to be "owned" by many persons and organizations in addition to the mental health center. This requires careful planning and the building of relationships.

Developing a Mental Health Education Program

Merrill Raber
Jane Hershberger

Prairie View and Its Catchment Area

Prairie View began in 1954 as a psychiatric hospital without any specific plans for preventive efforts in the community. Today Prairie View, a private nonprofit corporation located in Newton, Kansas, is a fully comprehensive community mental health center. The first federal grant was received in 1963. At that time the counties had the option of developing their own centers or contracting for services through Prairie View. Between 1963 and 1967, the three counties of Harvey, Marion, and McPherson all chose to develop contracts for services through Prairie View. These counties, located in the great plains of south central Kansas, have a total population of 78,000. The eastern portion of Marion County is located in Kansas' picturesque Flint Hills.

This tricounty catchment area of small town America is primarily populated by white, actively religious, and hard working people. The catchment area lies in what is known as the Bible Belt of America. This area was settled years ago by Mennonites emigrating from Europe and is still populated by many Mennonites as well as other mainline denominational groups. In Marion County there is a large population of Roman Catholics including a Czech

62

community. Blacks and Mexican-Americans make up a small portion of the population, especially in Harvey County. The Mexican-Americans moved into this area when laborers were needed for the development of the Santa Fe Railroad (the major industry in Harvey County) a century ago. There is substantial social and religious cohesiveness within the Mexican-American community that increasingly has an impact on the broader community. Traditional fiestas, annual statewide softball tournaments, community dances, and so forth are all participated in by the wider community. The current mayor of Newton is of Mexican-American descent.

In recent years there has been an increase in services to the black community and the Mexican-American community. The reasons for this are not clear, but, at least in the Mexican-American families, there has been less of the traditional prohibition against using resources outside the family and there is some suggestion that the mental health services are being seen as more available and more relevant to their needs.

The people in this area have unusual educational opportunities with six liberal arts colleges located here. These are all church related, having been established in the late nineteenth century. These colleges have developed a consortium known as the Associated Colleges of Central Kansas and currently are thriving in spite of a nationwide declining student population.

It is important to keep in mind the composition of the population of this area because the values of these actively religious people dictate in many ways the type of programming that Prairie View does. (See the chapters by Wagenfeld and Wagenfeld and by Giles in the present volume for a further discussion of values and service delivery.)

Origins of Community Involvement

During the early years, most of the community involvement was concerned with smoothing the way for referrals and helping reduce the stigma and misunderstandings concerning the role of mental health facility in a small, rural community. It was early in Prairie View's history, however, that groups referred to as religion and psychiatry study groups began flourishing as a result of efforts to communicate with the predominantly church-oriented community about the relationship between religion and psychiatry. This educational effort brought together a cross-section of the professional community and mental health professionals and became a significant bridge. In 1958, Prairie View began a conscious effort to become community oriented in its services. Philosophical underpinnings were gradually being evolved.

With the advent of national legislation in 1961 enabling the development of community mental health centers and the report of the President's Joint Commission on Mental Illness and Health, a major effort was underway at Prairie View to move from being a psychiatric hospital to what was to become known as a comprehensive community mental health center. It was in 1963 that a somewhat reluctant staff began setting aside several hours a week for increased experimental contacts in the community with public schools, juvenile judges, churches, and so forth. The reluctance was related to increasing pressure to provide clinical services but also to a lack of comprehension as to the concept of community-wide involvement and participation in the mental health enterprise.

By 1966 a director of consultation and education (C&E) was appointed and began to give approximately half time to the area of community involvement and development.

As more C&E activities developed, it became clear that the increased focus on these activities had not been coordinated with the change of treatment activities then being developed. A Department of Community Services was developed. This department merged both clinical and preventive tasks, with the agenda time of staff meetings divided between clinical and preventive issues. During this time (1968), the American Psychiatric Association awarded Prairie View the Gold Achievement Award, citing Prairie View for the transition from a psychiatric hospital to a comprehensive center. This transition included the beginning range of many C&E activities.

Although the number of C&E activities in the three-county area was significant, there was concern as to the theory base by which the activities were being developed. In the area of consultation, Gerald Caplan's model (1964) was perceived as the definitive approach. Staff members were increasingly aware, however, that the beginning consultation efforts in the community did not usually correspond to the systematic and formal consultation process that Caplan described as being appropriate. Also, about that time, the National Institute of Mental Health did a study/survey of consultation services being offered in mental health centers and visited Prairie View. This study (McClung and Stunden, 1970) confirmed that what was being done at Prairie View as a collaborative effort with other caregiving agencies was not only being done elsewhere but was also probably more appropriate in a rural mental health setting than was the more classic Caplan model. This study was also a turning point — allowing us to tie the activities more directly to some theoretical considerations — and a strengthening point in the efforts toward prevention.

Relationship of Consultation/Education and Prevention

Both the federal Community Mental Health Act of 1963 and the amendments of 1975 underscore the important role of educational services. But only recently has the public health model of primary prevention become a part of the community mental health center concept and lexicon.

The report of the President's Commission on Mental Health (1978) further established prevention as a major objective for mental health centers.

For a comprehensive rural mental health program, C&E become the vehicles for achieving the broader objective of prevention.

It is generally accepted that a broad concept of prevention includes not only the prevention of specific psychiatric disorders but also the positive promotion of mental health. It is the latter that becomes the main focus for C&E efforts in a rural mental health center. To promote this focus, not only a climate for healthful living must be created in rural communities but collaboration with other caregiving agencies as well. This collaboration needs to occur not only at the level of primary prevention but also at the secondary and tertiary prevention levels. This means that C&E become the first line of defense in a comprehensive center with twenty-four-hour hospitalization becoming the last resort after all other modalities have been exhausted. In a rural setting C&E activities must be organized in multiple ways that may be somewhat different from those required for an urban setting.

Basic Principles

Collaboration with Community Agencies. The principle of collaborating with other agencies becomes paramount in a rural setting. First, it is evident that many of the other caregiving agencies, such as schools, courts, welfare, public health, are often well-informed about the activities and effectiveness (or lack thereof) of each other's services. Other agencies in a rural setting respond best when mental health staff approach the task of working cooperatively with the many kinds of people in need. Frequently, those who are being seen at the mental health center are also being seen by other agencies as well. It is clear that the mental health center has not solved the whole problen, and this in turn gives the message to other agencies that mental health professionals do not have all the answers. Working together in this way mobilizes community resources that are urgently needed for effective results in a rural setting.

Use of Advisory Committees. Committees are often seen as difficult to manage, and advisory committees may be seen as unimportant and ineffectual. In a rural setting, however, the process of developing and maintaining multiple advisory committees is an important step in building community support. Advisory committees related to local finances are traditional. Advisory and satellite committees for giving feedback on educational needs begin the process of building both community ownership and staff accountability to the community. Committees can be built around various target groups, such as churches, families, industry, schools, and so forth. This process involves careful development and administration.

Building Trust. The first two principles discussed here speak to the development of trust. Further efforts to build trust can include the involvement of staff in community affairs, which typically means staff members need to live in the community where the C&E programs are being initiated. This process allows contacts with various segments of the community and conveys the message that the answers to mental health problems lie not so much in the mental health center as they do in the community. Developing a concept of partnership is a basic ingredient of success in the rural areas.

Needs Assessment. Both formal and informal assessment of needs occur in a continuing process of collaboration with a community. As a result, the mental health center increasingly cosponsors educational events with other interested groups in the community.

Use of Nonprofessionally Trained Staff. It is increasingly evident that people in the community who are not professionally trained in the usual mental health disciplines can sometimes be more effective in working with certain segments of the community than can the professionally trained staff, who often are encumbered with preconceived notions about interpersonal relations in a rural setting. Formal and informal training of selected people in the community can produce remarkable results. People who have received public welfare assistance can be most effective in working with other low income families, just as alcoholics often are most effective in working with other alcoholics. This also becomes a useful method of expanding the staff capabilities, but it is important to keep in mind that the trained staff needs substantial support to experiment with this idea.

Use of Adjunct Staff. The staff available for educational activities can be greatly expanded by making use of people in the professional and nonprofessional community who have special skills that can be marketed under the community mental health banner. Such people include college faculty, members of the clergy, homemakers, and others who have skills in specific areas and can be hired for specific events.

Building on Community Strengths. Most rural areas have a strong religious component. Developing special collaborative arrangements with members of the clergy and providing supportive services to churches may be a first step in relating to a major influence in the community.

Lighting Many Fires. Rural areas tend to mean scattered populations. Focusing on multiple ways to communicate with such scattered populations becomes critical to success. This includes finding ways to collaborate and to provide a variety of educational experiences to meet the multiple levels of readiness among the residents of the catchment area.

A large volume of growth-oriented events at a mental health center tends to create a milieu of prevention and health at the center rather than a climate of sickness. Over a period of time, a community begins to see a community mental health center as an educational institution in addition to being a treatment center. The concept of an educational center helps the staff deal with the stigma of mental illness and makes it possible for an increasing number of community members to feel comfortable about coming to the center.

This happens best when a fairly large volume of growth/educational events are offered at the center itself.

Involving the Community in Planning

To plan successfully and carry out the many mental health educational events in a catchment area, it is important to have a network of interested people who can help facilitate events. At Prairie View this network consists of a Family Life Education Advisory Committee in each of the three counties of the catchment area. One or two staff members meet with this group on a monthly basis for a two-hour lunch period. The meetings are held in each respective county.

The Family Life Committee determines through an informal process what kinds of mental health education programs are needed in each community for the coming year and helps with publicity and recruitment for these events.

The needs assessment is done by informal brainstorming at the monthly meetings. In addition to these monthly sessions, an annual meeting of all three Family Life Committees is held for half a day. At this time, committee members are encouraged to bring guests who might be interested in mental health education and can provide additional input. Such people are often invited to join a Family Life Committee.

In addition to the county-wide committees, satellite committees have been formed in a number of the small towns of each of the counties. The satellite committees are organized by Family Life Committee members representing that community. The committee members invite others interested in mental health education to a meeting at which a Prairie View staff member explains the program and asks for input and advice. These satellite committees are encouraged to meet once or twice a year or as needed to continue their planning and input for mental health education.

In general, the Family Life Committee members are enthusiastic about their involvement in the mental health programs and are eager to help promote health education in their community. They have begun to feel ownership of the Family Life Program as it is organized at Prairie View.

Frequently, as a result of the committee's involvement and investment, various educational events find multiple sponsors. This means that the actual brochure that goes out may have three to ten cosponsors for an event. These committee members also have been effective in recruiting for these programs.

Specific Kinds of Educational Events

The broadest categories of educational events can be identified as follows: public information; personal awareness; and intensive growth opportunities.

Public Information. The intent of public information programs is to communicate clearly and effectively the range of services available through the community health center. One of the most effective ways of introducing the public to services at a mental health center is by sponsoring an orientation event. At Prairie View, this has been done on Saturday afternoons and evenings, or on an evening only. Staff members have explained various aspects of the mental health center, including psychodrama, substance abuse treatment, and the admissions process, which is illustrated through role-play by staff members. At one of these events, the medical director explained how he and other staff members evaluate those who are brought to the mental health center for treatment.

The people invited to orientation events are primarily those who have some commitment to the promotion of mental health—for example, those who are already members of advisory committees such as the Family Life Education Committee and the Community Mental Health Services Advisory Committee, as well as volunteers and Board members. Each guest is encouraged to bring his or her spouse or another guest. Those attending are also invited to eat a meal in the center dining room.

Orientation acquaints people with services and staff members and promotes good will between them and the organization, as well as giving them an opportunity to ask questions about mental health services in a nonthreatening environment.

Health fairs are another effective public relations effort. At health fairs, displays that emphasize the educational services at a center rather than the treatment services also help to get the message across to the public that a mental health center is more than just a treatment center for the mentally ill. Because the mental health component is seen alongside other health components, mental health is put in the context of total wellness.

Prairie View has also used slide-sound sets as an effective public information tool. At Prairie View a separate slide set has been developed specifically for each of two of the three counties in the catchment area, as well as another slide set that includes the entire catchment area. Slide sets are frequently used with civic groups, church groups, planning meetings, or fund raising events.

Personal Awareness. Events that can be included in this category include both one-time presentations and ongoing workshops. Typically these one-time presentations consist of presentations and/or small group discussions about such selected mental health topics as stress, depression, or worry and may be presented to civic and professional clubs, senior centers, and nursing homes. Ongoing training groups and/or workshops offered to the public at large include assertiveness training, weight control, dealing with death and dying, coping with aging parents, and the relationship of physical fitness and mental health.

A good example of a personal awareness event is the class in weight control that has been held repeatedly at Prairie View. Recruitment for these classes is relatively simple because many people are concerned with their weight. Costs are kept low to allow as many people as possible to participate. Lay persons are recruited from the community to teach the classes. One is a home economist who is an expert in good nutrition and has in addition completed a behavior modification weight control class. She has gone on to use her experience and knowledge to develop a curriculum for teaching weight control. This community member has since trained another community person to teach the class, thus expanding the potential for offering classes in other communities. Although sometimes taught at the center, these weight control classes have also been held in outlying communities.

These classes convey the message that Prairie View is interested in providing a wide array of services to its catchment area and is also willing to bring the programs to the people instead of waiting for the people to come to Prairie View.

Parenting classes also tend to be nonthreatening in nature, so people are generally willing to enroll in them, especially since most people want to improve their parenting skills. For people living fifty miles away from the center, taking the class to the community often makes attendance possible and creates a new image of community mental health.

The use of entertaining films, such as *I Love You, Goodbye* and *Brian's Song*, can also be useful for leading discussions about mental health related issues. These films have been scheduled at as many as thirty locations within a two-week period, with various community leaders serving as discussion leaders.

Intensive Growth Opportunities. In this category are those in-depth events that may be more threatening but at the same time may help individuals to identify their particular needs. Such programs include marriage enrichment, workshops for divorced persons, and workshops on such topics as depression, stress, and relating to aging parents. In addition, men's and women's growth groups provide opportunities to discuss emerging role changes and the frequent fears and stresses that accompany these changes. An environment of trust helps lessen the reluctance to talk about these kinds of change and the problems that often result from them. It is from these groups, where the context is that of educational experience, that referrals for clinical services sometimes become appropriate.

Financing educational events in a community mental health center becomes a critical issue in an inflationary economy with increasing competition from other programs that offer similar kinds of programs. Obviously, it is important that financial considerations be carefully studied for the long-term continuation of educational mental health activities. At Prairie View, cost accounting has made it possible to identify the actual cost of the educational program. This means that salaries of staff who manage the C&E program are considered expenses as well as the overhead used by the deparment within the

Figure 1. The Scope of Mental Health Education in a Rural Community

	Mental Health Education	Mental Health Consultation	Training	Community Organization	Mental Health Promotion Groups
Schools/ Teachers	Life coping skills curriculum to integrate substance abuse issues with life experiences	To school counselors and referral liaison	In-service training for teachers		
	Worry clinics				
	Provide resource (mental health staff) for high school classes				
	One-day programs on sexuality in high schools				
	One-day programs on substance abuse in high schools				
	Films made available for loan to schools				
Employment Services	Assertiveness training for WIN clients	To employment service staff—case consultation	In-service for staff about substance abuse	Collaborate with First Step Industries in employment of youth	

Figure 1. The Scope of Mental Health Education in a Rural Community (continued)

	Mental Health Education	Mental Health Consultation	Training	Community Organization	Mental Health Promotion Groups
Churches/ Clergy	Values clarification program offered through churches and conducted by Prairie View (PV) staff	Consultation to West District ministers	Training of self-esteem and conflict resolution for clergy	Community service chaplain contacts made with every clergy person in catchment area	Clergy support group
		Staff available for free consultation with any clergy in catchment area	Self-directed learning for clergy continuing education		
	Sunday morning sermon and Sunday School classes focus on child abuse— conducted by PV staff	Consultation to clergy and hospital visitation	Stress management	Community service chaplain attends ministerial alliance meetings	
		To denominations in setting up support groups for clergy	Clergy and spouse marriage enrichment seminars	All pastors invited to visit PV center	
			Training for discussion group leaders in the church	Form an external advisory committee to PV's total services to churches	
				Hospital chaplain provides ongoing group consultation to pastors involved in community ministry	

Courts and Police		Community services chaplain available to police at any time for crisis situations	Train college personnel to provide services to prisoners	Monthly luncheon meeting arranged at PV for courthouse personnel involved in working with PV (both staffs review working relationship and mutual problems)	Families of prisoner's group meets regularly
Colleges	Staff available for convocations	Provide case consultation to faculty and students in six colleges		Ask for college faculty and staff to be on Family Life Education Committees	
Rape Victims		Home health agency care and organization To clients and staff of MidKap organization		Work with sexual assault team within county	Mothers' enrichment group
Industry		Employee assistance program Management training	Career development programs for groups and individuals Alcohol and drug abuse seminars Supervisory training	Monthly luncheon seminars provided at PV bringing together personnel from businss and industry (3 locations) Monthly luncheon meeting for case review	Women's growth group

Figure 1. The Scope of Mental Health Education in a Rural Community (continued)

	Mental Health Education	Mental Health Consultation	Training	Community Organization	Mental Health Promotion Groups
Nursing Homes		Case consultation Organization consultation	In-service programs on many types of subjects, such as emotional issues of aging, death, and dying		
Parenting	Positive parenting workshops				
Women	Growth groups; workshops with focus on women			Work with community battered women task force	Widows' support group
Aging	Workshops relating to aging parents, assertiveness for older adults, peer counseling		In-service training for nursing home staff		Over 60 groups
Other Mental Health Centers		Organization, development, and management training	Consultation skills training C&E training		
Couples	Marriage enrichment				
General Public	Workshops with one-shot programs— weight control, assertiveness training, holistic health, stress, depression				

total operation. The income includes federal, state, and local monies that can be applied to educational programs and the fees that can be charged for these services.

Charging fees is a complex issue since Prairie View is committed to providing services to everyone in the catchment area. In response to this issue, Prairie View has taken the stand that fee income should be expected whenever possible. This has required staff to think seriously, first, about the worthiness of any educational event being offered, and, secondly, about the philosophy involved in asking for fees. Educational events that do have a fee attached usually have some partial and full scholarships available. This is a way of recognizing the need for free service to some. Another way of managing this issue of fees is to have an internal public service fund that can be tapped for programs that the staff feel are urgently needed, when fee income would be insufficient to cover the cost.

The staffing pattern for C&E at Prairie View resembles a mixed model in that relatively few staff members are full time in C&E, while most of the staff are expected to provide some C&E time. C&E time needs to be monitored and coordinated for maximum effectiveness.

Another way of viewing our educational program is in terms of two dimensions — the type of activity and the target/population groups (see Figure 1). We can, for example, be concerned with what we have defined as mental health promotion, formal training, or consultation. These services can be provided to a variety of populations, such as other caregivers (school, social agencies, clergy) or "lay" groups. Mental health education for teachers, for example, might take the form of worry clinics or sexuality programs, while for groups of parents in the community we might run positive parenting workshops. Our training activities for clergy might be continuing education programs, while we might provide alcohol and drug abuse seminars for local industry. Our broad conception of the parameters of education and appropriate recipients or target groups enables us to respond to a diverse set of needs in the community.

In summary, the educational program is a concept that needs to be "owned" by many persons and organizations as well as the mental health center. In a rural setting this means giving maximum attention to building relationships with individuals and organizations throughout the catchment area, with a goal of creating a climate in which learning can take place.

References

Caplan, G. *Principles of Preventive Psychiatry.* New York: Basic Books, 1964.

McClung, F. B., and Stunden, A. *Mental Health Consultation to Programs for Children.* Rockville, Md.: National Institute of Mental Health, 1970.

President's Commission on Mental Health. *Report to the President.* Washington, D.C.: U.S. Government Printing Office, 1978.

74

Merrill Raber is director of the Growth Associates Division, and Jane Hershberger is coordinator of Consultation and Education at Prairie View Mental Health Center, Newton, Kansas.

As a microcosm of the community, the community mental health center itself becomes a laboratory for the study and examination of community mental health issues.

The Laboratory Approach to Community Mental Health Planning

P. Vincent Mehmel

The timely identification of and response to community needs may well be an essential ingredient in the successful development of a community mental health program. All too often, community mental health programs evolve amid high expectations and accompanied by an influx of new funding and a cadre of talented, enthusiastic mental health professionals in the absence of a realistic appraisal of what will be required to sustain this momentum. The degree to which such programs have been successful or unsuccessful may be closely related to the manner in which service implementation adheres to the conceptual framework for the program.

In evaluating the functioning of individual programs, attention should be given to all of the factors that are involved in a community mental health delivery system. However, the way in which programs are implemented and the interaction of the staff members with each other and with the community in this implementation does not always receive the attention that is warranted. Even when there has been active citizen involvement in the planning process and services are designed as a consequence of a careful needs assessment, there is no assurance that the resulting program will do what it is expected to do. The way in which a program is introduced and the professional staff's readiness and commitment to the task determine whether community needs have really been identified and addressed.

This chapter will give a few examples of how new programs have been introduced in response to community need in a rural community mental health program. Basic to the operation of this community mental health center (CMHC) is the belief that, within the professional staff of the CMHC, there should be reflected most of the attitudes, beliefs, and values of the community that the CMHC serves.

Currently, attention is being given to the governance issue of community mental health programs. Federal guidelines now require assurances as to the representativeness of the governing board and/or the advisory boards of these programs. Paradoxically this is occurring at a time when local governments are moving towards more direct administration of such public programs, ostensibly to make them more accountable to elected officials. It should be noted that the elected official is usually not elected to conduct a mental health program. It is also clear that elected officials may represent but are usually not representative of their constituency.

While community representation and involvement are important, they may be insufficient to sustain a quality program. Representativeness of the staff may be even more significant. Staff composition is usually looked at from the standpoint of professional qualifications, the presence of certain mental health disciplines, and minority representation. It may be equally desirable for staff composition of a comprehensive CMHC to reflect a cross-section of the community. Ideally, the social and cultural factors at work in the community should be present and manifest in the staff.

Although a CMHC is characterized by the multidisciplinary nature of the staff, the interdisciplinary mix is not always evident in the operation of specific program elements. This may be to the detriment of the program as a whole, as well as possibly limiting the impact of the individual service component.

With the possible exception of filling staff positions that are in short supply and hard to fill, selective factors are often at work in the recruitment process that interfere with the CMHC's ability to respond to community need. Such factors as age, experience, cultural and social background, among others, are approached with the view of building a professional team that is compatible and relatively homogeneous. The fact that this approach may constrict the program's response to community need is overlooked. Ideally, the staff of a community mental health center should be at least as diverse and heterogeneous as the community it serves. This diversity should include social diversity, occupational training, and diversity of experience. The commonality would be the specialized mental health training that has been received or is given and a commitment to the principles of community mental health. In CMHC settings where the staff is representative of the community or can be seen as a microcosm of the community, the CMHC itself becomes a laboratory for the study and examination of community mental health issues.

The Laboratory Approach to Programming

The laboratory approach to community health programming is particularly applicable in a rural catchment area. Distance alone precludes the easy establishment and proliferation of a particular service. Out of necessity a new program offering has to be phased in or introduced on a relatively small scale. This is very compatible with the building block design approach to the development of a comprehensive CMHC program.

The West Central Community Health Center in Willmar, Minnesota has endeavored to pilot almost everything before it is incorporated within the community mental health system. This applies to essential services, quality assurance mechanisms, as well as to office forms. This approach has a number of advantages. Among these are:
- An initial modest investment in resources (both staff and fiscal);
- Opportunity to observe staff and community resistance to a program while it is still a small-scale operation and develop an appropriate response;
- A capacity to work through "bugs" and logistical problems and modify the program accordingly;
- Opportunity to assess and develop staff skills and experiences within a new program offering and make the necessary adjustments;
- Staff team building;
- Opportunity to determine whether the anticipated use of the service will really be there and whether the full operation will be appropriate or adequate;
- A capacity to build in an evaluation component to assess whether the program will do what it is supposed to do.

To illustrate this approach, five examples will be given. These examples occurred over a period of twelve years. The examples are given not only to illustrate the pilot approach to introducing programs that are designed to respond to community need but also to give some indications of professional mental health staff response to new program initiatives.

Follow-Up Care Program. About twelve years ago, it was observed that the center psychiatrists' time was increasingly given over to medication control and supervision of chronically mentally ill patients. While these were essential services, they were for the most part the only services the chronically ill patient was then receiving in the program. It was suggested that perhaps another model of service delivery might be considered. While the concern over time involvement with existing practice was genuine, the willingness of the staff to do something new was limited.

Discussion ensued within the center program, and a pilot program was developed to serve these patients who, for the most part, had been discharged from the state hospital. It was evident that these patients could benefit from interaction with each other in a group setting close to where they lived. One of the psychiatrists, who was part-time, was interested in the opportunities such a program would provide for doing medication control in a group setting. A socialization program was also considered. Discussions were held with family service and public health nursing agencies in several of the counties served by the center. The reaction to the development of a cooperative program was mixed.

Nevertheless, a follow-up care program was designed that involved the building of an after-care team. This program was first established in a single county. Included on the team were a welfare caseworker, a public health nurse, plus a psychiatric nurse and a psychiatrist from the center. The service delivery model had the team working together in a group setting for a full half day in a community setting (for example, a church). The program provided for regular staffings, home visits, and crisis intervention, as well as socialization activities, group therapy, and group and individual chemotherapy. Evaluation of this program over the first year of its operation indicated its benefit for staff and patient. It was then initiated in other counties, where resistance to participation rapidly dissipated. It has been operational in all eight counties served by the center for a number of years.

Nursing Home Consultation Program. Within the consultation and education program of the center similar processes have occurred, as, for example, the development of the nursing home consultation program. Several stroke patients who were residents of nursing homes had been referred for rehabilitative services on an outpatient basis (speech therapy and occupational therapy). The provision of these services included the staff's visits to the nursing home. The resultant interaction of CMHC staff with nursing home patients and the staff of the nursing home made the need for preventive mental health services apparent. Several staff who had contact with nursing home patients and/or experience with nursing home settings got together to prepare a proposal for working with nursing homes. As a consequence of this proposal a nursing home consultation team was developed on a part-time basis to develop a consultation model for nursing homes. The initial team included a CMHC staff nurse (who had previous experience as a consultant to nursing homes and certification as a nursing home administrator), a speech clinician, and an occupational therapist. A no-fee contract was developed whereby members of the team made weekly visits to the nursing home to interact with patients and provide case and program consultation, including in-service training for nursing home staff.

The nursing home team accessed other CMHC staff (notably the pastor counselor and clinical psychologist) for special program offerings. Team members took refresher courses, attended specialized workshops, and visited other nursing homes to prepare themselves more fully for the challenges of this new program offering. This program was monitored and modified during the pilot year of operation. At the conclusion of that year, a nursing home consultation model had evolved that led to regular staff assignment to this activity and the development of year-to-year as well as ongoing consultation arrangements with a variety of nursing homes in the area.

Elderly Daycare Program. The success of the nursing home program has led to the development of a model for nursing home alternatives and the establishment of a daycare program that serves elderly clients within a twenty to twenty-five mile radius. Part of the original nursing home team has become involved in the inception of this program, while the nursing home consultation effort continues with some of the original staff.

Social Abuse Program. This program, a recent example of staff and community response to a current social issue, had its inception less than three years ago.

Some professional staff members working in inpatient and partial hospitalization programs were also involved in women's issues within the community. They became aware and concerned about the needs of women who were subject to abuse. Concommitant with their personal community involvement with this issue, they requested a needs assessment of this area within the context of their work situation. Their work assignment was modified to allow the needs assessment, which included a thorough survey of law enforcement and welfare agencies, hospitals, physicians, and clergy regarding the existence and extent of the problem. With this information and their community contacts, the staff members who had completed the assessment established a volunteer network of safe homes throughout a large geographical area. While these safe homes addressed a short-term need, they did not provide shelter and support for more than forty-eight hours. With administrative approval, the staff endeavored to work with the community to acquire a shelter. An older home, located in the major community of the area, was made available to the center by the county through a lease arrangement. Minimal remodeling was accomplished through a HUD grant, and the facility was furnished by volunteer donations.

Funding for the project was not immediately available, and only limited staff and other resources of the CMHC could initially be allocated. A good deal of voluntary effort went into the project both from center staff and the community. A variety of resources were used until stable funding support for the program could be realized. The "grass roots" movement was allied to the more traditional CMHC program and the ensuing product continues to reflect these varied influences. The Social Abuse Program now cuts across the overall operation of the center. In addition to the shelter and the safe house network, there are specialized programs for rape preventation and control in the consultation and education (C&E) program, in a batterer intervention program, crisis intervention, and other service components. The program, while still maintaining its "grass roots" quality, is an integral part of the comprehensive CMHC.

Adolescent Day Treatment Program. Our most recent example of a piloted program is the adolescent day treatment program. Originally, adolescents were admitted to the general psychiatric inpatient unit, where programming for them had to be adapted within modalities primarily directed toward an older adult population.

A youth drop-in program that had been operational provided an entry point into the CMHC network but did not provide the intensive intervention for which a significant number of adolescents had need. Although the temporary residence within the crisis intervention program responded to acute situations, unless these crises subsided to the point where outpatient services with scheduled family, group, and/or individual psychotherapy would be effective, the available programs were often inadequate. Outside the center system, referral would have to be made to specialized adolescent residential programs (usually long-term), or the adolescent might be taken up into the criminal justice system.

The need for an appropriate alternative had been identified in annual needs assessment surveys as well as in meetings with community caregivers. Schools, welfare agencies, clergy, courts, law enforcement agencies, as well as families, bewailed the lack of effective community alternatives.

In response to this need, a specific track for adolescents was designed within the day treatment program of the CMHC. It was felt that a model previsouly developed within the CMHC for outpatient primary treatment of alcoholics might lend itself for adaptation to the adolescent. This model provided day treatment intervention on a contractual basis with the client for a period of four weeks. The significant other was also involved in the program, and the program provided for weekly follow-up sessions over a two-month period before the treatment program could be considered completed. Since the evaluation studies of this program were encouraging, it was felt that it could be adapted for adolescents who were experiencing a relatively severe emotional disturbance.

The design favored the adolescent being at home throughout the treatment program. This was possible when he or she lived within daily commuting distance of the center. However, since the program would have to be accessible to the entire catchment area population, placement in a foster home for several nights during the week became necessary. The family service agency made the arrangements for such foster home placement and agreed to supervise it.

An educational component was also provided. An agreement was made with the local school district to provide a certified teacher of the emotionally disturbed, aides as necessary, and occupational therapy services. The teacher's responsibilities included (1) developing an individual educational plan; (2) identifying the adolescent's educational adjustment; (3) providing such remediation as possible during the treatment period; and (4) providing liaison and follow-up with the adolescent's home school.

The adolescent and the parents enter into a contractual treatment plan agreement at the time of intake. This requires full participation in the program, which also has provision for multifamily group therapy. The initial evaluation of the pilot model is encouraging but requires staff involvement at least equal to that in an intensive inpatient unit.

Staff involved in new programs are encouraged to visit places with similar programs, participate in workshops, and involve other staff in the program planning. Consultants are made available if indicated. Staff are subsequently involved in interpreting the program to the community and to agencies both within and without the catchment area.

At least during the pilot phase, it can be advantageous to use some of the existing staff of the CMHC. The staff involved have usually seen the need for the program being initiated, have generated enthusiasm for what is to be done, and know the community, its resources, and the people with whom they will have to relate. A new program provides a new challenge to their careers and fosters the growth and the development of the individual staff members.

Identifying community needs also necessitates knowing when a program can be implemented successfully. The need for the adolescent day treatment program, for example, was apparent for at least ten years. However, it became feasible only after other programs for adolescents had been initiated. Such residential programs as the adolescent unit at the state hospital, group homes, and drop-in programs seemed to be a prerequisite in this area. Moreover, the development of the adolescent program also required the prior establishment and mature development of the day treatment program at the center.

The staff of the center, as well as its citizen advisory groups, should be providing cues as to the timeliness of a new program venture. The sense of community should be present in the staff when viewed as a whole, despite the heterogeneity of its membership. Just because a particular program model has proven successful in other locales, it may not be replicable in a given area. Replication of the after-care program described earlier in this chapter has differed in each of the eight existing programs. The pilot phase helps this adaptation process. Even within small programs the piloting approach to the introduction of programs will help assure their assimilation and integration within the existing service network of the CMHC.

The Laboratory Approach in Rural Areas: Some Principles

Needs Assessment as a Continuing Process. With many new programs being developed simultaneously, needs assessment is sometimes done after the fact. When a careful needs assessment is done in a rural area, primary emphasis is usually given to the key informant approach.

This approach has some pitfalls. It is not difficult to obtain from potential referring sources an estimated number of people with whom they come in contact who have a particular problem and would benefit from a specialized program. Even when that number is accurate, it does not necessarily follow that the estimated number of referrals will result. This is particularly hazardous with respect to residential programs; existing treatment usages and referral patterns are likely to continue for some time, even when a new alternative program becomes available locally. It takes time to build client use, particularly in rural areas. The phase-in approach makes it possible to build the program without major expenditure and to assess whether the expected need does in fact exist and whether it will be sustained.

Other factors of needs assessment have relevance. Not all population groups will use a needed resource to the same degree or in the same way. A particular minority group with well-documented service needs may not make full use of a particular program. Special adaptations of the usual delivery system may be required. The adaptation might be in the staffing composition, the delivery site, the hours when a service is delivered, and so forth.

Response to the Fragmentation of Staff. Professional mental health staff working in a comprehensive CMHC are frequently expected to function as generalists. This may be attributed in part to the fact that diverse services have to be made available over a large geographic area. As a result, the professional mental health staff member has the opportunity (and often is expected) to provide a diversity of mental health services for which he or she may have limited preparation and sometimes limited interest. This can result in an unevenness of professional performance. In some instances it stimulates the professional to greater growth and development but in others it can have a stultifying effect. Symptomatic of the latter is the phenomenon of fragmentation.

The laboratory approach to community mental health programming can help address this problem. The introduction of a new service under the guidance of a highly qualified professional or with the promise of specialized training does much to reawaken the interest of the professional mental health staff person, whether or not he or she is initially involved in the new program. A climate of change can bring about cross-fertilization of ideas throughout the total program. The hard-pressed staff person can feel that an additional resource is available and, with that, additional supports. However, if it is felt that the new addition or service is taking away from existing resources and reducing the older care services of the program, new programs may be greeted with resentment. The attitude of the director of the overall program will be influential in determining the staff's reaction. He or she should not lose sight of the interdependence of staff growth and development with program growth and development.

Fiscal Integrity. Fiscal constraints can prevent the growth of mental health programs. They can also result in programs that are paper programs with little service capability. Either situation has a negative impact upon the credibility of the community mental health program. Through the piloting of a new service, the parameters of what is to be delivered are more carefully defined and the likelihood of overselling is reduced.

The piloting of a new program can be carried out on a restricted budget while providing an opportunity to assess what the true costs of the full program would be prior to a major outlay of funds. Piloting also makes it possible to appraise what the actual revenues will be and to work out the costly problems of delivery on a small scale. In rural areas the factors of time, travel, and coordination are particularly important logistical problems that have significant fiscal ramifications.

Time. A fundamental principle of community mental health is that the program become an integral part of the community. This is not achieved in a short period of time. Nowhere is this clearer than in a rural area. The laboratory approach, with its building block design, acknowledges this fact by the slow, inexorable development and modification of mental health service programs.

Legislators and study commissioners often overlook the fact that each task needs careful definition and a well-designed response. Each program element needs to be integrated into the community and within the total program. This is not easy to achieve, as the process is a dynamic one not unlike that which occurs within the development of the individual.

Evaluation. Despite the increasing attention given to evaluation in the past decade, it is a concept still not well understood. Moreover, it is unlikely that the definitive evaluation study is in the offing. This does not militate against evaluation but rather suggests that there is much to be said for a circumscribed approach to evaluation as against broad global assessments.

The laboratory approach to community mental health, particularly in a rural area, affords a unique opportunity for evaluation. A pilot study can allow for an evaluation component that may provide subsequent replication. The variables may be more readily identifiable and perhaps easier to control in a rural area. Unfortunately, the disposition for evaluation in a service-oriented program is not strong, especially when resources are limited. The availability of the necessary professional personnel is difficult to come by let alone to fund. Nevertheless, the opportunities are there and the potential dividends are great: The research and evaluation potential of the emerging rural community mental health program largely remains as an untapped resource.

*P. Vincent Mehmel, a psychologist, is director of the West Central
Community Mental Health Center, Willmar, Minnesota.
He has directed this comprehensive community mental health
in rural Minnesota since its inception in 1958.*

The small size and relative lack of complexity of the bureaucracy in a
rural state offers advantages to the mental health planner.

Rural Mental Health Planning: The Montana Experience

Peter S. Blouke
David Drachman

As a specific function of governmental agencies, planning is second only to regulation as the most justifiably maligned occupation of the bureaucracies. This is especially unfortunate in the field of human services, where vast sums are being spent on programs about which we have relatively little accurate data and even less understanding. This is not to say we do not plan; on the contrary, we plan, and plan, and plan *ad nauseum*. The basic problem is that too often the planners are functionally separated from the implementors. Or the implementors are not allowed (that is, forced) to participate in the planning process. As a consequence, budgets, politics, and the professional/personal biases that are a real part of the real world are left out of the planning process, and then we wonder why our carefully thought out and elaborately bound plan is quietly shelved in the interests of expediency. This chapter offers no universally applicable solution; rather we would like to present our experiences in a small rural state that—due to simple economics—serendipitously forces planners and implementors to interact. We will also discuss some of the factors that impact the planning process in a rural state.

Those engaged in mental health planning for heavily populated areas must often wish they could pursue their goals in a simpler environment with fewer agencies and clearer channels of communication. Rural environments, while in some respects simpler with regard to mental health planning, do pose several problems for the mental health administrator. Montana, with its large area (larger than all of the New England states combined) and sparse population (784,000 – 1978 estimate) certainly qualifies as a rural state. Contributing to its rural character is the absence of any concentrated urban areas: The two largest cities, Billings and Great Falls, each have approximately 60,000 residents. The economic and cultural foundations of the state are also rural: Logging, ranching, agriculture, and mining are the major industries.

As in other states, Montana has experienced a large exodus from the state psychiatric hospital in recent years. However, Montana has been more fortunate than most in that a reasonably comprehensive network of regional community mental health centers has developed that provides local services across the entire state and has been willing and able to absorb the deinstitutionalized population. The state's legislative and executive branches have been generous to mental health and, in 1978, Montana ranked sixth nationally in per capita expenditures for mental health services.

Responsibility for mental health affairs is vested in the Department of Institutions, Mental Health and Residential Services Division. This division has direct administrative authority for six state institutions: one for the mentally ill, two for geriatrics, two for the developmentally disabled, and one that serves alcoholics and drug abusers and also serves as a reservoir for overflow from other institutions. Additionally, the division has contractual responsibilities for the community mental health programs and two federal grants: a Mental Health Manpower Development grant and a Community Support Project. While there is line authority over the state institutions, the regional community mental health centers were established in 1975 by the legislature as private nonprofit corporations with whom the division contracts for mental health services. Currently, state funding for the centers is limited by law to 50 percent of their total budgets. It is through the budgeting process that the division impacts community mental health center (CMHC) programs and planning. Staff of the division includes an administrator, three staff, and clerical support. Staff responsibilities are divided according to community mental health, developmental disabilities, and institutional programming. There is no designated planner for the division.

Needless to say, the division is not allowed to function in a vacuum and its stewardship of mental health services is impacted by a host of other state and federal authorities. Compounding the task of state planning for mental health is the very nature of what we choose to define as mental health. Unlike energy or agriculture, which have reasonably discrete parameters for planning, mental health necessarily involves education, welfare, health, and housing authorities at every level of government – each promulgating overlapping and too often conflicting regulations. For Montana, the clearest current example is the debate over who has responsibility for the emotionally disturbed child. At least three different state agencies have broad statutory responsibility for assuring that mental health services are provided to this population. In addition to confusing the issues seriously, overlapping responsibility also allows for a considerable amount of old-fashioned passing of the buck. However, the local situation is crystal clear when compared to the federal regulations and interpretive guidelines associated with just P.L. 94–142 (Education for the Handicapped) and P.L. 94–63 (Community Mental Health Center Authorities). Unquestionably, the road to Hell was paved by governmental planning agencies.

In addition to its obvious rurality, Montana is also demographically small. An immediate and direct consequence of this is the firm conviction of our legislature that the central agency should also be of a corresponding size. Thus, despite our own best efforts to grow and multiply, the bureaucracy in Helena (Montana's capital) is relatively small and uncomplicated. This relative smallness impacts the planning process in several ways. Such a system is easy to comprehend, there is little difficulty in routing communications, and requests for assistance to the appropriate parts of the network are easily made. The system is further cemented by the many informal relationships that exist within and between agencies. The smallness of the bureaucracy also serves to concentrate the decision-making authority. While the size of the bureaucracy does not seem to have any beneficial effects on the length of meetings, the number of participants necessary to reach a decision is appreciably less than would be the case in a larger system. For example, the number of interagency personnel necessary to plan and develop jointly a cooperative group home for emotionally disturbed children was five. This is not to say that each agency official was so knowledgeable that considerable staff work was unnecessary. Rather, the individuals involved were close enough to the actual programs to appreciate the significance of their actions and vested with the necessary authority once a course of action was determined to make a decision and commit their agencies. Smallness also means that people must wear several "hats" and may be involved with a variety of different types of programs and populations. While at times confusing, such a small group of interagency personnel can assess the impact of a specific program across a wide spectrum of human services.

The size of the service delivery system itself also impacts the planning process. When a new program or direction is considered, a relatively small financial investment is needed for development of a demonstration project. For example, when we realized that Montana was not meeting its obligations to the emotionally disturbed child and consideration was given to development of a program that would fall somewhere between the tightly controlled environment of an institution and the typically unstructured community program, the project involved a single group home. Thus, using as a pilot project a group home involving eight to ten children per year, we can have a reasonable indication of the program's potential value for the entire system. In addition to the low cost of having only one such operation to monitor, the conception, planning, implementation, and evaluation phases are focused in such a manner that changes to the program can be made at any point without service disruption or delay. If the number of pilot homes necessary to evaluate the system had been six or seven, the process would inevitably have been much more complex and less amenable to ongoing adjustment. Additionally, by limiting the size of the project, it is relatively easy to keep everyone informed and involved throughout the planning and implementation process.

A less tangible, but also important, aspect of the size and informality of the system is that much of the jurisdictional jockeying that is often associated with interagency contacts can be eliminated. Although never fully understood by anyone, the operational parameters of different agencies can be learned to the extent necessary for negotiation of interagency planning, agreements, and contracts. The people involved become sufficiently familiar and comfortable with one another, so that much of bureaucratic game playing is eliminated.

Size is also a significant factor within the division. Because there is no designated planner, this function is shared by each member of the division. The annual state plan for comprehensive mental services, for example, is compiled by a single individual with input from every other member of the staff. Thus, those who will eventually be responsible for implementation of the plan are also those who write the plan. This assures that such factors as budget constraints, scarce manpower resources, and local politics are given consideration during the planning process.

By involving a variety of staff, a range of expertise and experience is brought into the process that would otherwise not be available: Staff members feel that they are more involved in the planning and decision-making process as it affects their own day-to-day operation. The fact that personnel who are actually involved in ongoing field operations are also involved in the planning process lends a certain amount of practical credibility to the document when it is received by the general public. In general, the final document is a realistic assessment of what can be accomplished.

Clearly, there are also significant drawbacks to such an arrangement. First, there is the risk that planning becomes an exercise to justify ongoing projects after the fact. Even with a very small staff, there is resistance to change and a normal reluctance to abandon programs or philosophies in which there are investments of time and energy. Thus, the inevitable frustrations that are experienced daily in any bureaucracy involved in human services can lead to a malaise that blunts the planning process. There is a value to detached, ivory tower planning that proposes what should be rather than accepts what is expedient. However, Montana cannot afford the luxury of a fulltime planner and necessarily must allocate existing staff to that function. In part, to offset any such tendency towards overreacting to pragmatic considerations, we have interpreted the federal guidelines requiring that the mental health agency council meet at least quarterly to mean they must meet at least four times a year. The council is a working group that only meets during the quarter when we are involved in development of the mental health plan. Thus, they are actively involved throughout the development of the plan and not asked simply to review a completed document during formal quarterly meetings.

A second potential weakness of nonplanner planning is that the planning process is given a low priority. In fact, this is true within our own division. The formal planning is done—that which is required by federal or state mandate—but little else in the way of long-range planning is accomplished. Specific projects, such as the children's program, are planned in the sense that a need is identified, a program conceived, and an implementation strategy developed; but we have yet to integrate this project into a comprehensive interagency plan for services to emotionally disturbed children. As we are reasonably sure is true in other states, the mental health agency has a state plan incorporating emotionally disturbed children, the state education agency has a state plan for services to emotionally disturbed children, and the state welfare agency has a plan incorporating services to emotionally disturbed children. We all know planning is important and should be a comprehensive effort and that sound planning will eventually reduce duplication and increase efficiency; too often, however, planning becomes lost in the rush to keep up with the pressures of day-to-day crises. Good planning is difficult and time consuming and crisis management is easier and more immediately gratifying than the drudgery associated with data collection, analysis, and writing. To the best of our knowledge, rural mental health agencies are as susceptible as urban agencies to this aspect of the planning process.

Finally, we would like to discuss some of the factors of rurality in Montana that impact the planning process. Our own experience indicates that the stereotype of the rural individual as an uninformed bumpkin, balking at change, living in a closed social structure, and clinging to old traditions is simply not true. In the smallest communities we have found a willingness to try new ideas. Except in very rare instances, the general public is no longer informationally isolated. The community leaders in rural Montana are just as informed about current events and trends as are the community leaders we have encountered in larger metropolitan areas. The advantage we enjoy is that, to swing a community's support behind a major project, fewer contacts with significant individuals are necessary to gain support and acceptance. The political structure of rural communities is certainly less complex and more personal than what might be found in a metropolitan area of over 50,000. As a general rule, to those who enjoy the intrigues and manipulations of bureaucratic game playing, rural community leaders and politicians may appear dull and unsophisticated. They have an annoying tendency to be direct, candid, and result oriented in their approach to new ideas and services. Rural communities are not receptive to mental health advocating major structural change in their community, nor do they believe it is the role of mental health to tamper with the community's value system. However, if the community is brought into the planning process at the beginning and the mental health services and benefits are explained, almost without exception mental health is encouraged and supported in rural areas.

The size of a community has another very significant impact on mental health planning as far as the economies of adding or subtracting a program are concerned. This factor becomes particularly relevant in relationship to the major state institutions and the process of deinstitutionalization. Montana's institutions were built during the days when "Out-of-sight, out-of-mind" was the cornerstone of mental health planning. The institutions are therefore located in rural areas and are a major employer for the surrounding communities. So far, Montana has not been faced with the prospect of closing any institutions but has had to deal with reduction in staffing. We have been fortunate that, during the period before deinstitutionalization, the low staffing ratios at the institutions mitigated wholesale reduction of staff as the populations decreased. Those who were appropriate for community programs have, for the most part, been transferred to the community. The residual population does require intensive psychiatric care in an institutional setting. We are cautiously optimistic that Montana has passed through its major thrust for deinstitutionalization and recognize that there is a very legitimate role for institutional programming for the mentally ill.

From an economic standpoint and due to the scarcity of professional resources, it has been necessary to centralize the more cost intensive services, such as partial hospitalization and group homes. As a result, there is a growing concentration of human service programs in the larger metropolitan areas. This is also true for other agencies, and competition is growing for location of mental health group homes, correction group homes, alcohol group homes, and developmental disabilities group homes. We are belatedly initiating the planning process to approach this problem of community saturation of agencies and hopefully can reach across our own immediate interest in service delivery to incorporate the planning and program development of other agencies.

Review of the most recent edition of the new Community Mental Health Systems Act, currently being considered by Congress, suggests that state mental health authorities may finally have the opportunity to control not only their own state funding sources but also the disbursal of federal funds. While this may have a certain amount of surface appeal by making it possible to regulate the proliferation of programs that ultimately demand state funding, there are inherent problems associated with such a relationship. In the absence of a clearly articulated and mutually agreed upon statement of the intent and responsibility of this tripartite relationship—local/state/federal—it is unlikely that truly effective long range planning or program stability can be accomplished. From the state's perspective and given the limits of fiscal resources, some very basic questions are being asked: Why is the state even considering funding CMHCs? What tangible results can be expected from these programs? What are the state's obligations and what should be local prerogative? What range of services does the local community want and to what extent is it willing to assume fiscal responsibility for these programs? What is the role of the federal government? Does the state want to obligate itself to long-range support of the multiplicity of programs mandated by the new Mental Health Systems Act? To say simply that we are jointly interested in improving the general mental well-being of the public or that we wish to continue the excellent programs currently in existence begs the question. Certainly the state has a responsibility to continue support of its deinstitutionalization program, but is there also a minimum service base that should be guaranteed by the state? If a local community wishes to provide marriage counseling, parent effectiveness training, rape counseling, or self actualization workshops, is this also a state responsibility?

To put it bluntly, control issues must be resolved. It is highly unlikely that state legislators are going to be willing to appropriate large sums to local programs without some very specific guidelines as to how that money should be spent. The state's beginning efforts to develop state-CMHC contracts for services to replace the current contracts have been given new impetus by this legislation because they offer a method for tying dollars to specific services performed. In Montana and, we would guess in other rural areas, a major strength of the current mental health system is its local identity and local autonomy. Where possible, decisions regarding services and service delivery mechanisms are made at the local level. We believe this aspect of the mental health system can and must be preserved. However, we also believe that its preservation is predicated upon a much clearer delineation of the specific roles, responsibilities, and expectations of the local, state, and federal partnerships.

Montana has been a rewarding professional experience for both authors. We have found that the advantages of rurality far outweigh the disadvantages in planning and development of mental health services. The willingness of people to work together cooperatively, the flexibility within the system, the multiple roles that must be played, and the immediacy of feedback for successes and failures more than compensate for the lack of sophisticated resources. Our system has problems, certainly, but somehow these problems seem much more amenable to resolution than those we imagine are found by the planners and implementors of program for large urban areas.

Peter S. Blouke is currently administrator of the Mental Health and Residential Services Division and David Drachman is program evaluator of the Community Support Project in the Montana Department of Institutions.

Attention to the mental health needs of rural Americans requires vigorous
and sustained advocacy. The development of this process at the National
Institute of Mental Health and some of its outcomes are described.

Rural Mental Health Programs and the Federal Government

Lucy D. Ozarin

This chapter describes an experience in advocacy for rural mental health at the
federal level. These advocacy efforts were directed toward agencies and their
component units to enlist their support and involvement in assuring that the
programs and funds they administered reached rural areas, a process that
required flexibility in administration and in interpreting regulations to meet
rural needs.

The National Institute of Mental Health (NIMH), part of a larger
component, the Alcohol, Drug and Mental Health Administration (ADAMHA)
of the Department of Health and Human Services (HHS) has responsibility at the federal level to carry out programs of research, personnel training,
and community services to promote mental health and prevent mental illness. The agency as directed by Congress provides leadership and direction to
the national mental health program through numerous grant programs and
provision of technical assistance.

NIMH, established in 1947 by an Act of Congress, had no identifiable
rural component until 1967 when, following a reorganization, a staff person
based in an applied research program was designated as a focal person for rural
mental health. As a result, extensive demographic and other data about rural

areas were collected, a small group of research grants were funded, and the beginnings of a communication network between rural mental health facilities were laid down.

In 1976, when the author was designated to serve as coordinator for Rural Mental Health, different external circumstances led to new directions and new approaches.

A basic question arose early: Should the rural mental health program seek to be a separate program with its own staff and budget, or should it seek to be part of all Institute programs? Because all programs in research, training, and community services apply to people everywhere, a decision was made not to opt for a separate rural component. Instead, the decision was to serve as an advocate for rural people, to raise the consciousness of all program administrators to rural needs, and to endeavor to ensure that rural areas received their share of available resources through flexible program administration and technical assistance.

Since, in a multiperson organization, one rarely can accomplish a large task alone, the need arose to enlist the aid of others with similar objectives and interests. A model used earlier had proved successful: The Community Support Program for Chronic Patients, started in one NIMH Division, had involved many divisions and other agencies and, after four years, had become a major program with its own staff and budget. The heart of this effort had been a work group with membership both from within and outside NIMH who could advocate for the program, serve as advisors, and provide input into planning. The model of a work group for rural mental health was adopted and membership solicited informally. For the past four years the group, which includes staff from most NIMH units, as well as other ADAMHA and Public Health Service agencies and the Department of Agriculture, has met regularly once or twice a month. The meetings allow exchange of information between members, information of a nature that might not otherwise be available. The work group meeting provides a forum for discussion of rural issues, and the members provide counsel and serve as a sounding board for the coordinator. Minutes of each meeting are written and sent to all work group members and others who have asked to be kept informed. The minutes were also sent to each of the ten HHS regional offices for the attention of ADAMHA staff. Feedback from regional staff indicates that the minutes are read. In addition, pertinent materials and news items dealing with rural mental health are appended to the minutes. Dissemination of information is a basic requirement for an advocacy effort.

Initially, requests for information about rural mental health programs from both inside and outside NIMH were channeled to the coordinator. Few materials were available, however. During the next few years, several information documents were prepared through personal service contracts at minimal costs. A monograph on rural mental health was prepared with a sixty-page overview article and 360 items in an annotated bibliography (Flax and others, 1979). Also, since transportation is recognized as a major problem in rural areas, the coordinator collected a large number of documents from the Department of Transportation and other agencies. A writer was obtained to prepare a monograph describing grant programs for transportation, results of demonstrations, where to seek assistance, and so forth (Allard, 1979). Other materials were collected from the literature and other publications. The dissemination of information effort was later to be formalized through a network building process to be described later in this chapter.

In order to receive more direct input from rural community mental health centers concerning their problems, a small meeting was held in 1977. About fifteen representatives of rural centers were invited, as well as several academicians and a state mental health program director. The two-day meeting focused on problems in administration, personal recruitment, and retention and research. Proceedings were published. This meeting highlighted problems that needed additional information and with some remaining funds, a small group of researchers in rural mental health were brought together to discuss issues. Again proceedings were published. Both proceedings were distributed widely.

Meanwhile, an opportunity arose to take advantage of an existing NIMH grant to the MITRE Corporation, a nonprofit group that carries out research for the federal government. The grant concerned the exploration of approaches to development and management of research. The rural mental health effort would provide a laboratory for the research.

Through a developmental effort involving the Rural Work Group (an ad hoc group drawn from agencies in the Public Health Service and the Departments of Agriculture and Transportation) and 200 rural providers and others concerned with rural mental health, five areas were identified as major obstacles in delivering mental health services in rural areas: transportation; personnel recruitment and retention; government rules and regulations; advocacy on the community level; interagency coordination.

To explore these five issues further, the MITRE Corporation held a small meeting in 1978, bringing together researchers and providers to identify and establish priorities for research. The report of the conference was published with the intent that the information might stimulate applications for research in the needed areas (Cedar and Salasin, 1979).

The MITRE conference highlighted the need to improve communication among all people concerned with rural mental health service delivery. Problems in one location may have found solution in another location, but the questions remained how information was to be channeled and innovations brought to attention. One approach was to recruit a small number of people who appeared to have put through successful innovations, to enlist their assistance in submitting descriptions of their programs. These descriptions are disseminated through a quarterly publication called *The Rural Connection* (for more information, contact Dr. John Salasin, METREK Division, MITRE Corporation, 1820 Dolley Madison Blvd., McLean, Va. 22101).

The activities in rural service delivery brought to light the special problems faced by minority groups in seeking and obtaining mental health services. Distance, sparsity of population, poverty, cultural perceptions of mental health and illness, and help seeking behavior all seemed to pose problems. With financial assistance from the NIMH Center for Study of Minority Problems, which had been drawn into the Rural Work Group, the MITRE group convened a small meeting of providers and researchers to focus on issues that required attention. Black, Hispanic, Native American and Asian representatives were present. A report of this meeting is in preparation and will help guide the advocacy efforts.

Still another effort in improving services for rural populations lies in a joint program with the Bureau of Community Health Services (BCHS), Health Services Administration (HSA). This bureau helps support about 1,000 primary health care and migrant clinics in medically underserved areas. About 70 percent of the clinics are located in rural areas. Funds from BCHS have supported over 100 grants to their health center grantees to forge a linkage with an accessible mental health facility, stationing a mental health professional in the health center with back-up from the mental health facility. The on-site mental health person provides consultation and in-service training to health center staff, screens and evaluates patients for mental health conditions, refers to the mental health agency when needed, performs triage and, in some cases, provides brief therapy. This linkage program begun in 1978 is now being evaluated. It may be noted that in 1976 the NIMH Rural Mental Health coordinator began to work with the BCHS, reviewing health center grants to determine how their programs might relate to CMHC programs and generally serving as a liaison between NIMH and BCHS in this area. The linkage and liaison activities now involve all three ADAMHA Institutes; formal agreements have been signed by the directors of HSA and ADAMHA and a variety of training efforts about alcohol, drug, and mental health problems are being projected for primary health care center providers through established training mechanisms.

The evolution of the rural mental health program described here was based on an advocacy effort. In a number of respects, it is still an advocacy program though facets, such as training of primary care providers, are now becoming institutionalized—that is, established and identifiable parts of existing, funded programs.

Two essential factors emerge from the experience. One is the role of information. Useful and important information must be received and must be disseminated. The greater number of channels for input and output, the more successful the advocacy effort. A second factor is the involvement of more and more staffs and programs, enlisting their participation in the efforts in whatever way can be found, looking for ways to make their programs grow in the process of providing more rural services. For instance, inviting the director of the Minority Center to make a presentation of his program to the Rural Work Group led to discussions resulting in his funding the Minority Conference described above. A new group whose participation is being invited is the NIMH Center for Work and Mental Health. Their attention has been drawn to the plight of migrant farm workers, a very underserved group from a mental health standpoint, with the hope and expectation that their work will include attention to rural needs.

Advocacy has many faces and many forms. It must be suited to the locale and the people whose concern and involvement is solicited, whether it be in a rural county or in a federal agency. Essential components include a driving force behind the effort, a constantly widening circle of support, and objectives that are acceptable to those whose support is sought.

References

Allard, M. A. *Rural Transportation for Human Services: A Guide for Local Agencies.* Washington, D.C.: Human Services Research Institute, 1979.

Cedar, T., and Salasin, J. *Research Directions for Rural Mental Health.* McLean, Va.: MITRE Corporation, 1979.

Flax, J., and others, *Mental Health and Rural America: An Overview and Annotated Bibliography.* Department of Health, Education, and Welfare Publication No. (ADM) 78-753. Rockville, Md.: National Institute of Mental Health, 1979.

Lucy D. Ozarin is assistant director for Program Development in the Division of Mental Health Service Programs of the National Institute of Mental Health. She has written extensively in the areas of hospital and community psychiatry. In 1980 she was the recipient of the American Public Health Association's Mental Health Section Award.

Index

A

Abnormality, as culturally defined, 4
Aday, L., 6, 10
Adolescents, day treatment program for, 80–81
Advisory committees, use of, 64
Alabama, Vietnam casualties from, 25
Alcohol, Drug and Mental Health Administration (ADAMHA), 93, 94, 96
Alcohol-related problems, in boom towns, 16–17
Allard, M. A., 95, 97
Alvarez, R., 6, 7n, 10, 11
American Medical Association, vii
American Psychiatric Association, x, 63
American Public Health Association, vii
Appalachia: program development in, 26–28; proportion of veterans from, 25; service barriers in, 27–28; treatment issue in, 30–31; values in, 7n, 26–27; veterans' outreach services in, 23–31
Aranda, P., 7n, 11
Arkansas, Vietnam veterans from, 25
Associated Colleges of Central Kansas, 62
Association for Rural Mental Health, vii

B

Bacon, F., vii, viii
Baumheier, E. C., viii, xi, 2, 10, 14, 21
Benedict, R., 4, 10
Bentz, W. K., 28, 31
Bernstein, B., 3, 10
Bi-State Mental Health Foundation: activities of, 54–55, 57–58; catchment area for, 51–52; conclusions from, 58–59; historical development of, 52–58
Blacks, values of, 7n
Blouke, P. S., xi, 37, 85–91
Boom towns: analysis of, 13–22; delivery challenges in, 18–19; human service needs in, 16–18; institutional changes in, 15–16; population growth impact on, 14–15; preimpact characteristics of, 14; and Wyoming Human Services Project, 19–20

Boulding, E., 22
Brodie, H. K. H., xii
Brooks, G. W., 34, 38
Brown, B., 7n, 12
Bureau of Community Health Services (BCHS), 96

C

California, Vietnam veterans from, 25
Campbell County, Wyoming, increased human service needs in, 18
Caplan, G., 63, 73
Carter administration, 24
Catchments, and delivery systems, 9–10
Categorical funding, problems with, 47
Caudill, H., 7n, 10
Cedar, T., 37, 38, 95, 97
Celenza, C. M., x, 39–49
Center for Study of Minority Problems, 96
Center for Work and Mental Health, 97
Chittick, R. A., 34, 38
Cleland, M., 24, 29
Cohen, J., 4, 11
Colorado, human service needs in, 17–18
Community agencies, collaboration with, 64
Community mental health center (CMHC): governance of, 76, 91; laboratory approach to, 75–83; staff of, 76–77, 81, 82
Community Mental Health Center Act of 1963 (P.L. 94-63), 40, 55, 63, 87
Community support, building of, 51–59
Community Support Program for Chronic Patients, 86, 94
Connecticut, Vietnam veterans from, 25
Cortese, C. F., 17, 18, 21
Craig, Colorado, increased human service needs in, 17–18
Culture, and delivery systems, 1–12
Cutler, D. L., 10

D

Davenport, J., 2, 10
Davenport, J., III, 2, 10

Spanish Speaking Mental Health Research Center, 7*n*

Spanish-speaking people: alternative delivery system models for, 6; and folk healers, 6, 7*n;* health service use by, 9; and perceptions of reality, 4–5; values of, 7*n*

Spring Lake Ranch, 34–36, 37

Srole, L., vii, xii

Staff: and community involvement, 53, 59; of community mental health centers, 76–77, 81, 82; for education program, 65; professional stimulation for, 37, 45, 46

Stenger-Castro, E. M., 5, 12

Stunden, A., 63, 73

Szasz, T., 4, 12

T

Third party payers, and deinstitutionalization, 36

Thomas, A., 7*n,* 12

Tischler, G. L., 10, 12

Torrey, E. F., 5–6, 7*n,* 9, 12

Training for living, concept of, 34

Trice, H., 4, 11

Trust, building of, 64–65

U

Uhlmann, J. M., ix, 13–22

U.S. Bureau of the Census, 2

U.S. Department of Agriculture, 94, 95

U.S. Department of Health and Human Services (HHS), 93, 94

U.S. Department of Housing and Urban Development (HUD), 15, 22, 79

U.S. Department of Transportation, 95

U.S. Region VIII Department of Energy, 14, 22

V

Values: in Appalachia, 7*n,* 26–27; concept of, 7, 9; confrontation of systems

of, 8; and delivery systems, 1–12; in rural areas, 7–9, 61–62

Vermont: deinstitutionalization in, 33–38; Vietnam veterans from, 25

Vermont State Hospital, 34

Veroff, J., 6–7, 8, 11

Vet Centers, 24–31

Veterans: readjustment problems of, 23–24; state proportions of, 25; treatment issue for, 30–31; Vietnam, outreach services for, 23–31

Veterans' Administration, ix, 24–31

Veterans Health Care Amendment Act of 1979 (P.L. 96-22), 23

Voluntary service program, and deinstitutionalization, 37

W

Wagenfeld, J. K., viii, 1–12, 37, 62

Wagenfeld, M. O., vii–xii, 1–12, 26, 31, 37, 62

Waldhern, S. A., 22

Wardwell, J. M., 21, 22

Weiss, R., xii, 11

Weisz, R., 18, 19, 22

Weller, J. E., 7*n,* 12, 26, 27, 31

Wells, M., 36, 38

West Central Community Health Center, 77–81

West Virginia: geographic barriers in, 8; values in, 27; Vet Center in, 28–30; Vietnam veterans from, 25

Willie, C. V., 7*n,* 12

Willmar, Minnesota, pilot programs in, 77–81

Wilson, J. P., 23, 31

Wisconsin, deinstitutionalization in, 33

Women: abuse of, 79–80; in boom towns, 16

World Health Organization, 34

Wyoming: human service needs in, 18; stress in, 19; Vietnam veterans from, 25

Wyoming, University of, 19

Wyoming Human Services Project, ix, 19–20

New Directions Quarterly Sourcebooks

New Directions for Mental Health Services is one of several distinct series of quarterly sourcebooks published by Jossey-Bass. The sourcebooks in each series are designed to serve both as *convenient compendiums* of the latest knowledge and practical experience on their topics and as *long-life reference tools.*

One-year, four-sourcebook subscriptions for each series cost $18 for individuals (when paid by personal check) and $30 for institutions, libraries, and agencies. Single copies of earlier sourcebooks are available at $6.95 each *prepaid* (or $7.95 each when *billed*).

A complete listing is given below of current and past sourcebooks in the *New Directions for Mental Health Services* series. The titles and editors-in-chief of the other series are also listed. To subscribe, or to receive further information, write: New Directions Subscriptions, Jossey-Bass Inc., Publishers, 433 California Street, San Francisco, California 94104.